Practical Transfusion Medicine
for the Small Animal Practitioner

The *Rapid Reference* Series

Books in the *Rapid Reference* series are ideal quick references, using a concise, practical approach to provide small animal practitioners with fast access to essential information. Designed to be used at a patient's side, these books make it easy to quickly diagnose and treat patients. With a spiral binding to lie flat, *Rapid Reference* books are an indispensable tool for the exam room.

Other *Rapid Reference* Series Titles

Life-Threatening Cardiac Emergencies for the Small Animal Practitioner
By Maureen McMichael and Ryan Fries

Two-Dimensional and M-Mode Echocardiography for the Small Animal Practitioner
By June A. Boon

Practical Transfusion Medicine for the Small Animal Practitioner

SECOND EDITION

Carolyn A. Sink MS, MT(ASCP)

Virginia Tech Animal Laboratory Services (ViTALS)
Virginia Maryland College of Veterinary Medicine
Blacksburg, Virginia, USA

WILEY Blackwell

This edition first published 2017 © 2017 by John Wiley & Sons, Inc

Editorial Offices

1606 Golden Aspen Drive, Suites 103 and 104, Ames, Iowa 50010, USA

The Atrium, Southern Gate, Chichester, West Sussex, PO19 8SQ, UK

9600 Garsington Road, Oxford, OX4 2DQ, UK

For details of our global editorial offices, for customer services and for information about how to apply for permission to reuse the copyright material in this book please see our website at www.wiley.com/wiley-blackwell.

Library of Congress Cataloging-in-Publication Data

Names: Sink, Carolyn A., author. | Preceded by (work): Feldman, Bernard F. (Bernard Frank). Practical transfusion medicine for small animal practitioner.
Title: Practical transfusion medicine for the small animal practitioner / Carolyn A. Sink.
Other titles: Rapid reference series (John Wiley & Sons).
Description: Second edition. | Ames, Iowa : John Wiley & Sons, Inc., 2017. | Series: Rapid reference series | Preceded by: Practical transfusion medicine for small animal practitioner / Bernard F. Feldman, Carolyn A. Sink ; photographs by: Donna L. Burton. | Includes bibliographical references and index.
Identifiers: LCCN 2016047602 (print) | LCCN 2016049038 (ebook) | ISBN 9781119187660 (pbk.) | ISBN 9781119187684 (pdf) | ISBN 9781119187677 (epub)
Subjects: | MESH: Blood Transfusion–veterinary | Blood Banks–organization & administration | Blood Specimen Collection–veterinary | Animals, Domestic | Handbooks
Classification: LCC SF919.5.B55 (print) | LCC SF919.5.B55 (ebook) | NLM SF 919.5.B55 | DDC 636.089/539–dc23
LC record available at https://lccn.loc.gov/2016047602

A catalogue record for this book is available from the British Library.

Wiley also publishes its books in a variety of electronic formats. Some content that appears in print may not be available in electronic books.

Set in 9.5/13pt Meridien by SPi Global, Pondicherry, India
Printed and bound in Malaysia by Vivar Printing Sdn Bhd

1 2017

This book is dedicated to veterinary professionals who are engaged in maintaining a viable and safe transfusion service.

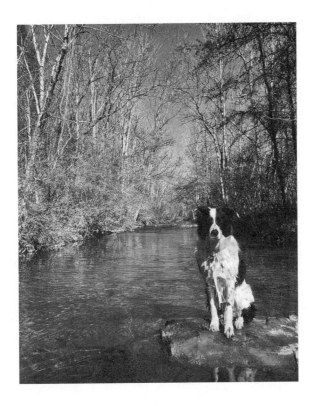

Contents

Preface

The scope of transfusion medicine encompasses blood donor selection, blood collection, processing and storage, pre-transfusion testing, blood transfusion therapy and outcome assessment. The ultimate goal is the proper use of blood and blood products in the treatment or prevention of disease. Interest in transfusion medicine by veterinary professionals surfaced at the 87th Annual Meeting of the American Veterinary Medical Association (AVMA) in 1950 and since this time, advances in human transfusion medicine have led to advances in veterinary transfusion medicine, as blood bank techniques and transfusion therapy protocols are improved and easily adapted for use in the veterinary field. *Practical Transfusion Medicine for the Small Animal Practitioner*, 2nd edition, is a comprehensive and concise guide for veterinary professionals who participate in any aspect of transfusion medicine and who wish to ensure the overall quality of the service.

Blood donor procurement and maintenance of a viable and safe donor pool is detailed. An overview of blood collection techniques is highlighted, and blood collection systems are reviewed, with an emphasis on popular configurations used for veterinary blood products. Blood anticoagulants and red cell preservatives are explained to assist the reader in producing safe and efficacious components that benefit the recipient.

Practical Transfusion Medicine for the Small Animal Practitioner, 2nd edition, contains detailed methods on how to fractionate whole blood into blood components; storage guidelines are included. Laboratory considerations in transfusion practice, including blood typing and crossmatch procedures are presented. Summarized charts are provided as testing guides when appropriate. Physiologic principles and indications for whole blood and component transfusion are described, along with assessment of transfusion outcome.

About the Companion Website

This book is accompanied by a companion website:

www.wiley.com/go/sink/transfusion

The website includes:
- Color images of the figures provided in the book.

Chapter 1 The Blood Donor

Introduction

Blood donors are vital to the success of any transfusion service, and veterinary blood banks depend on qualified donors to provide the blood necessary to meet the needs of the patients they serve. Donors may be a part of an in-clinic or community-based program, but to attract and maintain owner participation in either program it is essential that the blood donor qualification and donation process be as organized, pleasant, and convenient as possible. Established methods to produce safe products and maintain donor health are essential.

Owner Recruitment

Enlisting owners to volunteer their pet as a blood donor can be as simple as expressing the need. This can be done by mentioning the need for blood donors to clients or could include utilizing social media, websites, and posting notices in the lobby of veterinary clinics. Whether the donor will be part of an in-clinic or community-based program, many veterinary blood donor programs offer incentives to owners as compensation for time spent scheduling donations, transporting their pet to and from donations, or any other related activity (Table 1.1).

Good communication is imperative to the success of any blood donor program, and it is beneficial to define and communicate owner expectations during the blood donor qualification process. Suggestions for the contents of a written participation agreement can be found in Table 1.2. Standardized forms should be completed for enrollment of potential blood donors (Wardrop *et al.*, 2016); see Tables 1.3 and 1.4. Organizing staff members to coordinate and oversee donor recruitment, blood collection, and donor maintenance will streamline and contribute to the overall effectiveness of the blood donor process.

Practical Transfusion Medicine for the Small Animal Practitioner, Second Edition. Carolyn A. Sink.
© 2017 John Wiley & Sons, Inc. Published 2017 by John Wiley & Sons, Inc.
Companion website: www.wiley.com/go/sink/transfusion

Table 1.1 Incentives to recruit and maintain veterinary blood donors

Free donor vaccines
Free or discounted initial and annual blood donor physical exam
Blood product discount for participants
Dog spa or overnight boarding discount
Grooming services
Free or discounted pet food and/or treats

Table 1.2 Blood donor owner expectations

Obligations and benefits of the blood donor program are pending until the animal is accepted into the program

The owner agrees to bring the donor to phlebotomy location at the scheduled time for x times per year and once per year for the annual blood donor examination

At the end of the year if total number of donations does not exceed x or if the owner withdraws the animal before making at least x donations, the owner may be billed for the general physical exam and blood testing

If a donor's temperament is too difficult for continued phlebotomy on more than one occasion or if the owner is deemed uncooperative, the owner will be notified of their removal from the program. The owner will not be billed for any previous physical exams or blood tests relating to the blood donor program

The physical examination and laboratory tests necessary to qualify and maintain the animal as a blood donor are performed at no cost to the owner

Animals whose physical examination or laboratory results reveal a need for further diagnostic testing and/or medical treatment will not be accepted into the blood donor program. The owner may reapply to the blood donor program after the animal is declared healthy

The owner agrees to use year-round (12 months a year) monthly heartworm and flea preventatives that are approved by the blood donor program (if applicable)

If the cat is housed with dogs or if fleas are noted on the cat at any time, the owner agrees to use year-round (12 months a year) monthly flea preventative approved by the blood donor program as long as the cat is active in the program (if applicable)

Donors will receive annual vaccinations, heartworm preventative and flea/tick prevention treatment products at no cost for as long as they remain in the program (if applicable)

Source: Virginia Maryland College of Veterinary Medicine Teaching Hospital (2012).

It is important to select owners who are interested in the blood donor program and who understand their pet's participation in the program truly saves lives. Conscientious owners will be helpful in maintaining and monitoring the overall health status of the donor so that neither the blood donor nor the blood supply is compromised in any way.

Donor Attributes

While exact donor requirements vary between established blood banks, animals should be healthy and possess an agreeable temperament.

Table 1.3 Canine donor selection criteria questionnaire

Owner name
Dog name
Date
Is your dog between 1 and 8 years old?
Does your dog weigh more than 50 pounds (lean body condition)?
What is the breed of your dog?
Do you give your dog heartworm, flea and tick preventatives year round?
If the response is no, are you willing to give these preventative year round?
Has your dog been vaccinated in the past 12 months for distemper, parvovirus, leptospirosis, hepatitis?
Is your dog currently vaccinated for rabies?
Is your dog on any medications including NSAIDs, aspirin, vitamins, herbals?
Has your dog tested positive for Lyme disease?
Has your dog ever received a blood or plasma transfusion?
Has your dog ever been pregnant?
Are you aware of any health problems in your dog?
Do you travel with your dog?
Has your dog, its parents or siblings had a bleeding problem?
Are you staying in this area for the next 1–2 years?
Are you willing to drop the dog off at the hospital at no charge for the day?
Are you comfortable with a 3-inch area of hair to be clipped from your dog's neck for each blood draw?

To be completed by clinician or technician:
Does the dog resist being placed on an examination table?
Does the dog attempt to bite?
Does the dog have a readily accessible jugular vein?
Does the dog resist being restrained for jugular venipuncture for 3 minutes?
Does the animal resist being restrained in lateral recumbency for 2 minutes?
Does the dog resist venipuncture of the jugular vein?
Is the dog a likely candidate for the blood donor program?

Source: Virginia Maryland College of Veterinary Medicine Teaching Hospital (2012), Wardrop *et al.* (2016).

Canine Blood Donors
Physical Attributes

Males and non-pregnant females between the ages of 1 and 8 years old who have never had a blood transfusion are ideal blood donors. Clinically normal dogs can donate between 15 and 22 ml of whole blood per kilogram (kg) of body weight every 4–6 weeks without need for iron supplementation (Brown and Vap, 2012; Gibson and Abrams-Ogg, 2012; Schneider, 1995). In order to utilize conventional blood collection systems designed for humans (450 ml whole blood capacity), dogs should weigh at least 23 kg (in lean body condition). To facilitate blood collection and to maintain an aseptic phlebotomy site, donors should possess readily accessible jugular veins that lack thick skin and neck folds. Donors should be calm in nature so that vascular trauma is minimized and so that blood donations can be performed in less than 10 minutes with minimal restraint.

Table 1.4 Feline donor selection criteria questionnaire

Owner name

Cat name

Date

Is your cat between 1 and 8 years old?

Does your cat weigh more than 11 pounds (lean body condition)?

What is the breed of your cat?

Has your cat been vaccinated in the past 12 months for feline viral rhinotracheitis, calicivirus, panleukopenia?

Is your cat currently vaccinated for rabies?

Is your cat on any medications including NSAIDs, aspirin, vitamins, herbals?

Has your cat ever received a blood or plasma transfusion?

Has your cat ever been pregnant?

Are you aware of any health problems in your cat?

Do you travel with your cat?

Has your cat, its parents or siblings had a bleeding problem?

Are you staying in this area for the next 1–2 years?

Are you willing to drop the cat off at the hospital at no charge for the day?

Are you comfortable with a 2″ area of hair to be clipped from your cat's neck for each blood draw?

Are you comfortable with sedation and/or anesthesia of your cat?

To be completed by clinician or technician:

Does the cat have a readily accessible jugular vein?

Is the cat friendly and easy to handle?

Is the cat a likely candidate for the blood donor program?

Source: Virginia Maryland College of Veterinary Medicine Teaching Hospital (2012), Wardrop et al. (2016).

Utilizing donors who require sedation is discouraged unless exceptional circumstances prevail (Gibson and Abrams-Ogg, 2012).

Vaccination status should be current. Donors should not be receiving any drug therapy, although dogs should be given flea control treatment and those living in heartworm endemic regions must receive prophylaxis.

Laboratory Evaluation

Every blood bank should establish appropriate laboratory testing to qualify blood donors into their donor program. Normal levels of coagulation factors, hemogram and biochemical profile results, along with negative fecal and heartworm disease tests support healthy donor status. Donors should be screened for blood-borne pathogens. The American College of Veterinary Internal Medicine (ACVIN) Consensus Statement (Wardrop et al., 2016) contains an in-depth discussion of both optimal and minimal standards for appropriate blood-borne pathogen testing for canine and feline blood donors in North America; minimal standards for dogs are summarized in Table 1.5. The Consensus Statement also contains recommendations for laboratory evaluation of disease endemic to a particular geographic location.

Table 1.5 Recommendations for laboratory evaluation of canine blood donors for blood-borne pathogens

Minimal standard	Agent
PCR negative	*Babesia canis vogeli*
	Babesia gibsoni
	Bartonella henselae
	Bartonella vinsonii var. *berkhoffi*
	Mycoplasma haemocanis
PCR negative or *no screening*	Other *Babesia* spp.
PCR negative or seronegative	*Ehrlichia canis*
PCR negative or seronegative if serologic testing is more	*Anaplasma phagocytophilum*
economical or yields a more rapid turnaround time than PCR	*Anaplasma platys*
PCR negative in high-risk areas; *no screening in low-risk areas*	*Ehrlichia chaffeensis*
PCR negative or seronegative in high-risk areas, *no screening*	*Ehrlichia ewingii*
in low-risk areas	
PCR negative and seronegative in high-risk dogs; *no screening*	*Leishmania donovani*
in low-risk dogs	

PCR, polymerase chain reaction.
Source: Data from Wardrop *et al.* (2016).

Table 1.6 Importance of canine blood groups in veterinary transfusion medicine

Incidence of the blood group antigen in the recipient population
Incidence of naturally occurring antibody or antibodies against a particular blood group antigen
Presence of alloantibody due to previous exposure (i.e., transfusion)
Effect of naturally occurring or alloantibody against the antigen during transfusion

Source: Hale (1995).

During the initial blood donor qualification screen, the donor's blood type should be assessed.

Canine Blood Types

The importance of canine blood groups related to veterinary transfusion medicine is listed in Table 1.6.

Dog blood groups were among the first to be recognized in species other than humans. Early studies recognized that dogs do not have clinically important naturally occurring antibodies, so subsequent experimentation focused on alloantibodies produced after sensitization via blood transfusions (Swisher and Young, 1961) and led to international recognition of seven blood groups termed dog erythrocyte antigens (DEA) (Blias *et al.*, 2007).

Unfortunately, because of the limited availability of blood typing reagents it has not been determined if the currently recognized blood groups are

Table 1.7 Dog erythrocyte antigens

Canine blood group	Antigen phenotypes	Incidence in US	Presence of naturally occurring antibodies
DEA 1.0	1.1	45%	<2%
	1.2	20%	
	1.3		
	Null		
DEA 3	3	6%	<15%
	Null		
DEA 4	4	98%	Rare
	Null		
DEA 5	5	10–15%	8–12%
	Null		
DEA 6	6	100%	Unknown
	Null		
DEA 7	7	40–55%	10–40%
	7′		
	Null		
DEA 8	8	20–40%	Unknown
Dal	Dal	93%	Rare

Source: Hale (2012, 1995).

serologically distinct (Blias *et al.*, 2007). Likewise, the biochemical properties and molecular genetics of dog blood group systems are yet to be thoroughly investigated or well defined (Hale, 1995), so additional canine blood groups will likely be identified as immunohematologic technology improves and new antigens are discovered (Blias *et al.*, 2007).

The DEA canine blood group system is based on eight antigens found on canine erythrocytes (Hale, 2012). These blood groups are inherited independently so more than multiple antigens can be present or absent on the red cells of a given donor. Currently, only DEA 1.1 blood type can be easily identified using point-of-care testing. Six DEA blood groups can be distinguished utilizing more complex laboratory methods but two DEA blood groups can no longer be recognized because of the lack of commercially available antibody.

The current designation for DEA or blood type uses the numeral to indicate positive status. For example, "DEA 1.1,7" indicates that dog red cells express DEA 1.1 and 7 but do not express DEA 3, 4, and 5. When typing for DEA 1.1 only, the blood type is indicated as DEA 1.1-positive or DEA 1.1-negative (Hale, 2012).

A summary of DEA blood groups can be found in Table 1.7.

DEA 1

The DEA 1 system consists of three antigens (1.1, 1.2, 1.3) and a null phenotype. The subtypes of DEA 1 likely result from the difference in the number of antigen molecules on the surface of the red blood cell and variation in the biochemical composition of the antigen (Hale, 2012). DEA 1.2 antigen appears to be recessive to 1.1 so only a dog that is 1.1 negative can be 1.2 positive (Acierno *et al.*, 2014; Hale, 2012).

DEA 1.1 is the most commonly identified dog blood type but varies among breeds and geographically. Along with 1.2, it is highly antigenic. DEA 1.2 recipients who are transfused with DEA 1.1-positive cells can develop 1.1 antibodies, so dogs that are DEA 1.2 (or 1.3) positive should be transfused with DEA 1.1-negative cells. DEA 1.0 system is most often associated with acute immunological transfusion reactions in dogs.

DEA 3

This antigen has a higher incidence in American-bred greyhounds and Japanese-bred dogs (Hale, 2012). It can be found in only 6% of dogs in the United States and approximately 20% of DEA 3-negative dogs possess naturally occurring anti-DEA 3 (Hale, 1995). Anti-DEA 3 alloantibodies produced as a result of a previous transfusion can cause a delayed transfusion reaction (5–7 days post transfusion), which is significant in transfusion management of patients with non-regenerative anemia (Hale, 2012).

DEA 4

As up to 98% of all dogs are DEA 4 positive and naturally occurring anti-DEA 4 is not reported (Hale, 1995), acute and delayed transfusion reactions have been reported as a result of alloimmunization to DEA 4 (Metzler *et al.*, 2003) but statistically these transfusion reactions rarely occur. This is the only DEA blood group that a "universal donor" possesses.

DEA 5

DEA 5 is another rare canine blood group that occurs in approximately 10–15% of the general population. Approximately 10% of the dog population possesses naturally occurring antibodies to DEA 5. Transfusion of DEA 5-positive cells to a sensitized recipient can lead to a delayed transfusion reaction 5–7 days post transfusion, which is significant in transfusion management of patients with non-regenerative anemia (Hale, 2012).

DEA 7

Unlike the DEA systems described above, DEA 7 not an integral erythrocyte membrane antigen; the antigen is found in circulating plasma and passively attaches to surface of the red blood cells.

DEA 7 is present in 40–55% of the general canine population and naturally occurring anti-DEA 7 is present in 20–40% of DEA 7-negative dogs (Hale, 2012). Low incidence of delayed transfusion reactions has been reported, while acute transfusion reactions are yet to be documented. Because of the potential for delayed transfusion reaction, DEA 7 status plays an important role in compatibility for transplants or massive blood transfusion.

Selection of Blood Type for Blood Donors

Dog erythrocyte antigens and the prevalence of antibodies against specific DEA antigens should be considered when selecting donors. For transfusion services that supply blood products to clinics in which the majority of transfusions are expected to be once-in-a-lifetime occurrence, the inclusion of all canine blood types in the donor pool may be appropriate (and will broaden the donor base). Conversely, if most recipients are expected to need multiple transfusions or are candidates for transplantation, it may be appropriate to only include specific blood types in the donor pool to in an effort to decrease recipient exposure to foreign red cell antigens.

Feline Blood Donors

Like their canine counterparts, feline blood donors should be friendly and clinically normal.

Physical Attributes

Cats are typically sedated for phlebotomy and can donate between 10 and 12 ml of whole blood/kg body weight every 3–4 weeks (Kohn and Weingart, 2012). They may be supplemented with iron as appropriate. Collecting up to 50 ml of whole blood from a healthy, lean donor weighing more than 5 kg is usually safe (Kohn and Weingart, 2012), but blood donation is not without serious risk so appropriate client communication is essential when qualifying donors. Both males and females can be utilized and only current pregnancy excludes females (Abrams-Ogg, 2000); previously transfused cats should be excluded if alloimmunization has occurred. Cats should be between the ages of 1 and 5 years old and vaccines should be up to date. Strictly indoor cats are preferred so that the risk of disease transmission is minimized. Any other cat within the same household must be 100% indoor and appropriately vaccinated. Flea control should be administered if the potential donor is housed with dogs.

Laboratory Evaluation

Normal levels of coagulation factors, hemogram and biochemical profile results, along with negative fecal and heartworm disease tests support healthy donor status. The ACVIN Consensus Statement (Wardrop et al., 2016) contains an in-depth discussion of both optimal and minimal standards for appropriate blood-borne pathogen testing for feline blood donors in North America; minimal standards are summarized in Table 1.8. The Consensus Statement also contains recommendations for laboratory evaluation of disease endemic to a particular geographic location.

Table 1.8 Recommendations for laboratory evaluation of feline blood donors for blood-borne pathogens

Minimal standard	Agent
PCR negative	*Bartonella henselae*
	Mycoplasma haemofelis
PCR negative or seronegative if serologic testing is more economical or yields a more rapid turnaround time than PCR	*Anaplasma phagocytophilum*
Antigen negative	Feline leukemia virus
Antibody negative	Feline immunodeficiency virus

Source: Data from Wardrop *et al.* (2016).

Table 1.9 Cat blood groups by geographical locations

Location	Group A (%)	Group B (%)	Group AB (%)
Australia	62	36	1.6
Japan	90	10	0
United Kingdom	67.6	30.5	1.9
United States (by region):			
Northeast	99.7	0.3	0
North Central	99.4	0.4	0.2
Southeast	98.5	1.5	0
Southwest	97.5	2.5	0
West Coast	94.8	4.7	0.5

Source: Day (2012), Andrews *et al.* (1992).

Blood type should also be determined during the initial blood donor evaluation.

Feline Blood Types

The feline AB blood group system includes types A, B, and AB. The AB blood group system is controlled by three alleles and characterized by the type and amount of neuraminic acid present on red cells. An additional feline blood group antigen, *Mik*, has also been identified (Weinstein *et al.*, 2007). Feline blood types are geographically related as outlined in Table 1.9.

Cats possess naturally occurring alloantibodies which are formed against the A or B red cell antigen the cat lacks; type AB cats possess no naturally occurring alloantibodies. When present, alloantibodies can be responsible for transfusion reactions and neonatal isoerythrolysis. Anti-A alloantibody in type B cats is usually of high titer and is believed to be induced by exposure to cross-reactive environmental antigens within the first three months of life after maternally derived antibody is degraded. Anti-A alloantibodes are mainly IgM and cause acute transfusion reactions within seconds of transfusing type A or type AB red cells to a type B cat.

Anti-B alloantibody in type A cats is uncommon and, if present, is invariably of low titer (Day, 2012).

Existing outside the AB system, naturally occurring anti-*Mik*, present in cats lacking the *Mik* antigen, can elicit an acute hemolytic transfusion reaction after an AB matched blood transfusion.

Blood Donor Selection

Qualification of veterinary blood donors utilizing the criteria outlined above should be repeated at least annually (less the donor's blood type) and allows the clinician to evaluate physical exam and laboratory test findings in view of the overall goals of the blood donor program. More frequent retesting for some blood-borne pathogens in endemic areas and in donors with repeated exposure to risk factors may be necessary to insure the safety of the donor pool.

Initial and annual blood donor exams do not eliminate the need to perform a physical exam and minimal lab work prior to phlebotomy.

In human blood banking, donor eligibility is based on medical history and limited physical examination on the day of phlebotomy. Individual units of blood are screened for evidence of infectious disease pathogens for every blood donation. While this protocol is yet to be economically feasible for veterinary blood banks, it remains a gold standard.

Donor Monitoring

Once donors are qualified into the blood donor program, it is necessary to track essential information regarding individual donors, including vaccination status, last annual checkup, and last phlebotomy date.

Scheduling Donors

Contacting owners in advance or placing donors on a routine schedule can be a convenient method to schedule donors for phlebotomy. When contacted, owners should be queried regarding any changes in the donor's health status since the last office visit or blood donation. A standardized pre-phlebotomy questionnaire including any questions that may pertain to any change in health status, such as recent weight loss, acute vomiting or diarrhea, or change in behavior is helpful in accomplishing this task; see Tables 1.10 and 1.11.

Table 1.10 Pre-phlebotomy questionnaire for canine blood donors

Since your dog's last blood donation, has your dog:

Had any health problems?
Received a blood or plasma transfusion?
Been in any fights or received any bites?
Been sexually active or become pregnant?
Been on a raw diet?
Have you noticed fleas or ticks on your dog?
Have you traveled with your dog?

In the 48 hours after your dog's last blood donation, did your dog:

Resume a normal activity level?
Experience any diarrhea, vomiting or lack of appetite?

Today, is your dog:

Acting normal?
Receiving heartworm, flea and tick preventative?
Taking any medications other than heartworm, flea and tick?
Fasting?

Source: Virginia Maryland College of Veterinary Medicine Teaching Hospital
(2012), Wardrop *et al.* (2016).

Table 1.11 Pre-phlebotomy questionnaire for feline blood donors

Since your cat's last blood donation, has your cat:

Had any health problems?
Received a blood or plasma transfusion?
Been in any fights or received any bites?
Been become pregnant?
Been outside?
Have you noticed fleas or ticks on your cat?
Have you traveled with your cat?

In the 48 hours after your cat's last blood donation, did your cat:

Resume a normal activity level?
Experience any diarrhea, vomiting or lack of appetite?

Today, is your cat:

Acting normal?
Receiving heartworm, flea and tick preventative?
Taking any medications other than heartworm, flea and tick?
Fasting?

Source: Virginia Maryland College of Veterinary Medicine Teaching Hospital
(2012), Wardrop *et al.* (2016).

References and Further Reading

Abrams-Ogg A. (2000) Practical blood transfusion. In: *BSAVA Manual of Canine and Feline Haematology and Transfusion Medicine*. Day MJ, Mackin A, Littlewood JD, eds., pp. 263–303. Gloucester: British Small Animal Veterinary Association.

Acierno MM, Raj K, Giger U. (2014) DEA 1 expression on dog erythrocytes analyzed by immunochromatographic and flow cytometric techniques. *J Vet Intern Med* 28: 592–598.

Andrews GA, Chavey PS, Smith JE. (1992) Production, characterization, and applications of a murine monoclonal antibody to dog erythrocyte antigen 1.1. *J Am Vet Med Assoc* 201: 1549–1552.

Blias MC, Berman D, Oakley DA, Giger U. (2007) Canine Dal blood type: a red cell antigen lacking in some Dalmatians. *J Vet Intern Med* 21(2): 281–286.

Brown D, Vap LM. (2012) Principles of blood transfusion and crossmatching. In: *Veterinary Hematology and Clinical Chemistry*, 2nd edn. Thrall MA, ed., pp. 205–222. Ames, IA: John Wiley & Sons.

Day MJ. (2012) Feline blood groups and blood typing. In: *BSAVA Manual of Canine and Feline Haematology and Transfusion Medicine*, 2nd edn. Day MJ, Kohn B, eds., pp. 285–288. Gloucester: British Small Animal Veterinary Association.

Gibson G, Abrams-Ogg A. (2012) Canine transfusion medicine. In: *BSAVA Manual of Canine and Feline Haematology and Transfusion Medicine*, 2nd edn. Day MJ, Kohn B, eds., pp. 289–307. Gloucester: British Small Animal Veterinary Association.

Hale AS. (1995) Canine blood groups and their importance in veterinary transfusion medicine *Vet Clin North Am Small Animal Practice* 25(6): 1323–1332.

Hale AS. (2000) Canine blood groups and blood typing. In: *BSAVA Manual of Canine and Feline Haematology and Transfusion Medicine*, 1st edn. Day MJ, Mackin A, Littlewood JD, eds., pp. 281–288. Gloucester: British Small Animal Veterinary Association.

Hale AS. (2012) Canine blood groups and blood typing. In: *BSAVA Manual of Canine and Feline Haematology and Transfusion Medicine*, 2nd edn. Day MJ, Kohn B, eds., pp. 280–283. Gloucester: British Small Animal Veterinary Association.

Kohn B, Weingart C. (2012) Feline transfusion medicine. In: *BSAVA Manual of Canine and Feline Haematology and Transfusion Medicine*, 2nd edn. Day MJ, Kohn B, eds., pp. 309–318. Gloucester: British Small Animal Veterinary Association.

Metzler KJ, Wardrop KJ, Hale AS, Wong VM. (2003) A hemolytic transfusion reaction due to DEA 4 alloantibodies in a dog. *J Vet Intern Med* 17(6): 931–993.

Nusbaum RJ. (2013) Supporting an in-house veterinary blood bank. Western Veterinary Conference. Las Vegas.

Schneider A. (1995) Blood components collection, processing, and storage. *Vet Clin North Am Small Animal Practice* 25(6): 1245–1261.

Swisher SN, Young LE. (1961) The blood grouping systems of dogs. *Physiol Rev* 41:495–520.

Virginia Maryland College of Veterinary Medicine Teaching Hospital. (2012) Blood Bank Policies and Procedure Manual (unpublished).

Wardrop KJ. (2007) New red blood cell antigens in dogs and cats – a welcome discovery. *J Vet Intern Med* 21:205–206.

Wardrop KJ, Reine N, Birkenheuer A, Hale A, Hohenhaus A, Crawford C, Lappin MR. (2005) Canine and feline blood donor screening for infectious diseases. *J Vet Intern Med* 19: 135–142.

Wardrop KJ, Birkenheuer A, Blais MC, Callan MB, Kohn B, Lappin MR, Sykes J. (2016) Update on canine and feline blood donor screening for blood-borne pathogens. *J Vet Intern Med* 30: 15–35.

Weinstein NM, Blias MC, Harris, K, Oakley DA, Aronson LR, Gieger U. (2007) A newly recognized blood group in domestic shorthair cats: the *Mik* red cell antigen. *J Vet Intern Med* 21(2): 287–292.

Chapter 2 Blood Collection

Introduction

Blood collection in dogs and cats necessitates careful planning to minimize potential donor reactions or contamination of the unit of blood. For dogs, specialized equipment can facilitate and expedite blood collection; for cats, specialized blood collection systems are needed so that blood can be processed for storage. Product need, use, and storage should be evaluated prior to blood collection so that the appropriate collection system and anticoagulant are used.

Basic Equipment Needs

Blood Collection
Canine
Canine blood collection is outlined in Table 2.1.

Vacuum, Chamber, and Scale
A chamber attached to a vacuum source facilitates blood flow into the blood collection bag, thus reducing the amount of time that the donor must be restrained. The clear plastic chamber is cylindrical and one end is capped; the top has a lid. The blood collection bag is positioned within the chamber by means of a hook fastened to the removable lid; a small-notched opening at the top of the cylinder allows egress for the primary blood collection tubing (Figure 2.1). Once an empty blood collection system is placed inside the chamber, the entire apparatus is placed on a gram scale, which serves to monitor the weight of the blood bag during collection. The vacuum source is attached to the chamber by an inlet (Yagi, 2016) and low pressure is initiated prior to venipuncture.

Practical Transfusion Medicine for the Small Animal Practitioner, Second Edition. Carolyn A. Sink.
© 2017 John Wiley & Sons, Inc. Published 2017 by John Wiley & Sons, Inc.
Companion website: www.wiley.com/go/sink/transfusion

Table 2.1 Procedure for dog blood collection

Supplies needed
- Prep containers
- Dry gauze
- Blood collection system
- Vacuum chamber
- Vacuum source
- Gram scale
- Clamp
- Tube stripper
- Metal clamps and clamper

Procedure

1. Hang the blood collection system from the hook on the lid of the vacuum chamber. When the chamber is capped, the integrally attached needle, along with ample length of tubing, should run through the notched opening (at the top of the chamber) to exit the chamber. Make sure there is enough slack in the line inside the chamber to allow the bag to fill. The line should not be occluded.
2. Clamp the line a few inches back from the needle and set aside. This helps to prevent air from entering bag when the needle cap is removed.
3. Place the vacuum chamber on the gram scale.
4. Securely restrain and place the dog on a table in right lateral recumbency with the neck extended to gain access to the left jugular vein. The front legs may need to be pulled back slightly (to move the shoulders out of the way).
5. Clip the fur and prepare the phlebotomy site using aseptic technique. Sterility of the venipuncture site should be maintained at all times.
6. Turn the vacuum on and verify the pressure is not over 4 mmHg. Tare the gram scale to zero.
7. Remove the cap from the needle. The phlebotomist may palpate and puncture the skin adjacent to the jugular vein before advancing the needle into the vein. Remove the clamp from the phlebotomy line.
8. If blood is not free flowing, pinch the tubing clamp site open before repositioning the needle.
9. Encourage the donor during blood donation.
10. Monitor the gram scale to ensure the blood is flowing at a reasonable rate. The blood collection should take between 5 and 7 minutes, with a maximum of 10 minutes. Clamp the phlebotomy line when the appropriate blood volume is collected and remove the needle from the jugular vein.
11. Attend to the venipuncture site.
12. Turn off the vacuum and remove the blood collection system from the chamber. Remove the needle by clamping the line near the needle and cut the needle free.
13. Strip the blood from the phlebotomy line into the primary bag at least three times.
14. The product is ready for processing.

Sources: Melanie Gevedon, personal communication (2016), Gibson and Abrams-Ogg (2012).

Tube Stripper

A tube stripper is used to push or "strip" blood from the donor tubing into the primary blood collection bag. Starting at the sealed end from which the needle was removed, tubing is placed between the two Teflon™ rollers of the stripper. Once the tube stripper is engaged, the tubing is pulled through and away from

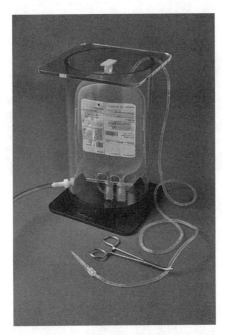

Figure 2.1 Proper set up of blood collection bag within vacuum chamber. Source: Animal Blood Resources International. Reproduced with permission.

the stripper while the tube stripper is pushed towards the primary blood collection bag (Figure 2.2). By continuing to occlude the donor tubing with the rollers of the stripper, blood that was formerly in the tubing can be mixed with the anticoagulant in the primary container. Once the occlusion created by the tube stripper is released, anticoagulated blood is returned to the donor tubing, which can be sealed to produce segments (representative whole blood samples of the unit). Alternatively, this process can be accomplished by manual rolling the donor tubing (Gibson and Abrams-Ogg, 2012).

Sealer

Sealers are used to both contain the blood product and to impede contamination of the blood product. This can be accomplished by use of electric heat sealers or hand sealers using metal clips (Figures 2.3 and 2.4).

Feline

A vacuum, chamber, and scale can be used in feline blood collection, although vacuum pressure via syringe is the most popular phlebotomy method. A tube stripper and sealer are also needed (see above). Feline blood collection is outlined in Table 2.2.

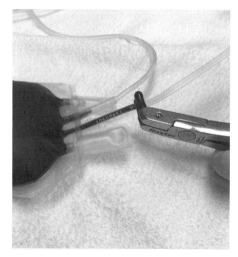

Figure 2.2 Tube stripper, used to return or "strip" blood from the collection line into the primary blood bag.

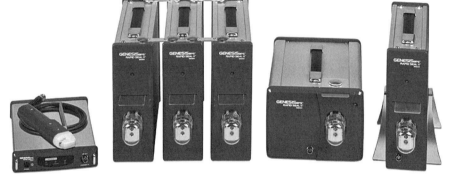

Figure 2.3 Tube sealers. Source: GenesisBPS. Reproduced with permission.

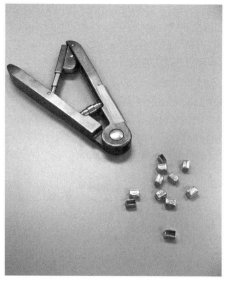

Figure 2.4 Hand sealer and metal clamps.

Table 2.2 Procedure for cat blood collection

Supplies needed

- 60 ml syringe
- 7.5 ml CPDA
- 19 gauge butterfly catheter
- 3-way stopcock (if storing blood for later use)
- Clippers with #40 blade
- Betadine® scrub
- Isopropyl alcohol
- 4×4 gauze sponges
- Vet wrap
- Sedation
- Lacri-lube®
- Exam gloves

Procedure

1. Sedate the cat:
   a. Ketamine (5 mg/kg) with midazolam (0.2 mg/kg): add midazolam to ketamine syringe immediately prior to intramuscular injection. Peak effect is not immediate; wait 20 minutes before evaluating need for additional drugs
   b. If ketamine/midazolam fails to sufficiently sedate the cat for phlebotomy, administer 55–100% of the same dose of ketamine with intravenous midazolam or use isoflurane delivered in 100% oxygen through a mask to immobilize the cat.
2. Position cat in sternal or lateral recumbency.
3. Apply Lacri-lube® to both eyes.
4. Shave hair over jugular vein and scrub 3 times with Betadine® scrub; wipe with alcohol after each scrub
5. Draw 7.5 ml CPDA (1 ml CPDA per 7 ml blood; reduce volume if less blood is needed) into 60 ml syringe and attach to butterfly catheter.
6. Nick the skin if it is tough prior to venipuncture. Puncture the jugular vein and gently withdraw blood until the syringe is full (52.5 ml blood + 7.5 ml CPDA = 60 ml total for a standard "feline unit"). Gently rotate syringe during collection to facilitate anticoagulant–blood mixing.
7. Remove the needle from the jugular vein and apply digital pressure to the neck for several minutes, then wrap the neck using a 4×4 gauze pad and vet wrap.
8. Administer 100–125 ml of 0.9% saline or lactated Ringer's solution subcutaneously to donor cat. Observe until fully recovered.
9. Product is ready for processing.

Sources: Melanie Gevedon, personal communication (2016), Kohn and Weingart (2012), Virginia Maryland College of Veterinary Medicine Teaching Hospital (2012).

Whole Blood Separation

Centrifuge

Because red blood cells, plasma, and platelets have different specific gravities, separation of whole blood into components is best accomplished by using differential centrifugation. When selecting a centrifuge, the bag size and the type of product(s) that will be centrifuged should be considered. The centrifuge

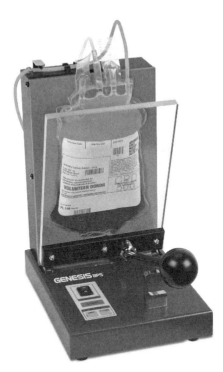

Figure 2.5 Plasma expressor. Source: GenesisBPS. Reproduced with permission.

bucket must be adequate in size and shape to house a full unit of blood plus any satellite bags that accompany the blood collection system. If fresh whole blood is processed into red blood cells and plasma, a refrigerated centrifuge with a temperature range of 1–6°C is needed. Additionally, rotor size, centrifugation speed, and duration of speed should be considered. Rotor heads with swinging buckets provide a level red cell meniscus and allow for maximum plasma recovery (in contrast to centrifuges with fixed rotor heads that produce an angled meniscus.)

Plasma Extractor

A plasma extractor is used to express plasma and plasma components from red cells. After centrifugation, the primary blood bag is placed between a fixed stainless steel and movable transparent plate which is spring loaded. Once unhinged, the transparent plate applies pressure to the blood bag and plasma is expressed into a satellite bag, as seen in Figure 2.5.

Scale

A scale for weighing blood products, both during and after blood collection, is needed to estimate product volume.

Blood Storage

The ability to store blood and blood products improves efficiency of blood collection and transfusion by eliminating the need for donor-to-recipient, vein-to-vein transfusion. Refrigerators and freezers are utilized to store blood and blood products, ensuring the availability of safe and effective blood products for transfusion.

Refrigerator

Refrigeration is crucial to protect the efficacy of blood and blood components. Whole blood and red cell products are stored between 1 and 6°C. Since the required storage temperature must be maintained at all times, a method to continuously monitor refrigerator temperature is ideal. Shelves or drawers assist in product segregation and inventory management. Emergency power back-up may be necessary if electrical complications frequently arise.

Freezer

Blood plasma is processed into a variety of components that have stringent storage requirements to preserve the clotting factors. Once separated from whole blood, plasma is rapidly frozen and stored at −18°C or below. Since the product must be maintained frozen, a method to continuously monitor the freezer temperature is ideal. Freezers with time- and temperature-dependent defrost cycles can be utilized as long as the defrost cycle does not excessively warm the product and compromise product viability.

Anticoagulant–Preservatives and Blood Collection Systems

Blood obtained for transfusion can be collected and prepared using a variety of anticoagulants, anticoagulant–preservative or anticoagulant–preservative–additive solutions; many bag configurations are commercially available. Evaluation of the collection system and anticoagulant requires knowledge of product shelf life; selection of a particular blood collection system is based on transfusion needs of the clinic or patient (Waldrop, 1995). Therefore, prior to blood collection, product need should be assessed to determine the anticoagulant–preservative and blood collection system best suited to product need (Table 2.3).

Table 2.3 Anticoagulant–preservatives and red cell shelf life

Anticoagulant–preservative	Contains	Red cell shelf life at 1–6°C
ACD	Anticoagulant–citrate–dextrose	21 days
CPD	Citrate–phosphate–dextrose	21 days
CP2D	Citrate–phosphate–double dextrose	21 days
CPDA-1	Citrate–phosphate–dextrose–adenine	35 days

Anticoagulant–Preservative Solutions and Red Cell Additives

Anticoagulant–Preservative Solutions

Anticoagulants prevent blood from clotting, and blood collection systems utilize liquid solutions contained in the primary bag. The anticoagulant used for blood collection directly impacts product integrity and maintains the unit of blood in a liquid, transfusable state.

Sodium citrate is the most commonly used anticoagulant; its action is to sequester calcium ions *in vitro*. Preservatives are phosphate-dextrose solutions, which prevent detrimental changes to the red cells by maintaining pH and promoting adenosine triphosphate (ATP) production (Table 2.4). The combination of anticoagulant–preservative provides a safe environment to store blood products: red cell products should be stored between 1 and 6°C, plasma products at −18°C or lower, and platelets at 22–25°C.

Anticoagulant–preservative solutions are not bactericidal. Refrigeration of red cells and freezing plasma products assists in inhibiting microbial growth within the blood product.

Red Cell Additives

Nutrient red cell additives are used in addition to anticoagulant–preservative solutions and increase red cell survival beyond that of an anticoagulant–preservative used alone. Additives are added to the red cells remaining in the primary blood bag after most of the plasma has been removed. This allows recovery of maximum amounts of plasma. Since the additive solution is directly added to the red cells, the final hematocrit of the red cell component is approximately 60%, which allows for excellent transfusion flow rates and eases blood administration. Additives must be added to red cells within 72 hours of collection.

There are four commercially available additive solutions: Adsol®, Nutricel®, Optisol®, and SOLX®. The constituents of these additives vary by manufacturer, but all contain dextrose, adenine, and sodium chloride. Other constituents

Table 2.4 Components of anticoagulant–preservative solutions and their action during blood storage

Component	Action
Citrate	Acts as an anticoagulant: chelates calcium and inhibits several calcium dependent steps of coagulation cascade
Dextrose	Nutritional support for red blood cells: supports ATP generation through glycolytic pathways
Phosphate	Optimizes pH for red blood cell survival (substrate for 2,3 DPG production): 2,3 DPG levels maximize oxygen release from hemoglobin to tissues
Adenine	Nucleotide substrate pool for ATP synthesis by the RBCs

Table 2.5 Constituents of red cell additives

Additive	Contains	Red cell shelf life at 1–6°C
AS-1 (Adsol®)	Dextrose, adenine, mannitol, sodium chloride	42 days
AS-3 (Nutricel®)	Dextrose, adenine, sodium phosphate, sodium chloride, sodium citrate, citric acid	42 days
AS-5 (Optisol®)	Dextrose, adenine, mannitol, sodium chloride	42 days
AS-7 (SOLX®)	Dextrose, adenine, sodium phosphate, mannitol, sodium bicarbonate	42 days

Source: American Association of Blood Banks (2013).

that may be included are sodium phosphate, mannitol, sodium citrate, and citric acid (Table 2.5).

Shelf Life

A unit of blood is a biosystem; death is innate. The stored or "banked" product has a specific shelf life, which is based on functional considerations of the blood product and also determined by the properties of the anticoagulant–preservative.

The shelf life of a blood product is the maximum allowable storage time.

Length of storage time is also affected by the configuration of the blood collection device: whether it is an open or closed system.

Closed System

Closed blood collection systems are designed so that the only opportunity for the bag or its contents to be exposed to the external environment is during venipuncture. Closed systems have integrally attached needles connected to satellite bags that contain anticoagulant–preservative–additive solutions. Using a closed blood collection system, sterility of the blood and blood products is not compromised during collection or processing into components for storage.

Closed blood collection systems have an expiration date independent of product collection dates. This expiration date guarantees anticoagulant–preservative–additive and bag sterility. The system expiration date is printed on the blood bag or the secondary overwrap (manufacturer packaging used for multiple bag purchase). Blood bags are single packed in a polypropylene bag and sterilized in the packaging, which helps ensure sterility prior to use. The polypropylene bags are packed in a secondary overwrap package, usually aluminum foil. Follow the manufacturer's guidelines for the expiration date of unused blood collection systems as the viability of the remaining unused blood bags is limited once the secondary overwrap is opened. Some bag configurations are available individually packaged.

Open System

An open system lends itself to increased probability of product contamination during collection, processing, and storage, as there are multiple opportunities for introducing contaminants. Open systems include syringes, bags without integrally attached collection needles or satellite bags. Blood collected in an open system must be used within 4 hours of collection if the product is stored at 22–25°C or 24 hours if stored at 1–6°C.

Blood Collection Systems

A wide variety of blood collection systems are available for both canine and feline blood collection.

Canine Blood Collection Systems
Open Systems
Syringes or empty collection or transfer bags with anticoagulant added at the time of phlebotomy are classified as open systems.

Historically, heparin has been used as an anticoagulant in open systems. Heparin acts as an anticoagulant by accelerating the action of antithrombin III, neutralizing thrombin, and preventing the formation of fibrin from fibrinogen. Heparin also deactivates platelets, making its use prohibitive for collection of blood for treatment of coagulation disorders. Heparin does not provide nutrients to facilitate red cell survival and is not recommended for routine blood collection and storage.

Citrate-containing anticoagulant–preservatives are preferable to heparin. Sodium citrate acts as an anticoagulant by chelating calcium. When used alone, sodium citrate is not suitable for collection of blood for transfusion because of its pH. Citrate used in conjunction with dextrose is the anticoagulant of choice for collection of blood for transfusion because it has a low toxicity and is easily metabolized.

Closed Systems
Human blood collection systems can be used for dog phlebotomy (Figure 2.6). Anticoagulant–preservatives include ACD, CPD, CPDA-1, and CP2D. ACD, CPD, or CP2D used in a closed collection system allows for red cell shelf life of 21 days when stored at 1–6°C. CPDA-1 allows for red cell shelf life up to 35 days when stored at 1–6°C. Additives extend red cell shelf life up to 42 days.

Feline Blood Collection Systems
Open Systems
The volume of blood drawn from a cat blood donor is considerably less than its canine counterpart. A typical feline donation is approximately 50 ml, making

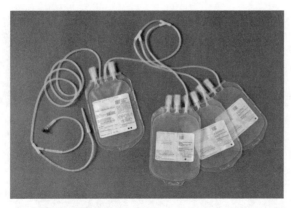

Figure 2.6 Quad blood bag used for canine phlebotomy. The additional satellite bags allow plasma to be divided into smaller volume units. Source: Animal Blood Resources International. Used with permission.

60 cc syringes a popular blood collection device. Since this is an open system, blood stored at 1–6°C should be used within 24 hours of collection.

The anticoagulant of choice is ACD, CPD, or CPDA-1 (Kohn and Weingart, 2012). The volume of the blood drawn is critical since too little blood with too much free citrate is contraindicated in cats. Citrate not consumed in anticoagulation is a notable chelator of patient calcium, so much so that severe and often delayed hypocalcemia can occur. CPDA-1 anticoagulant (1.2 ml CPDA-1 per 8.8 ml blood) is far superior to any other commonly used anticoagulant, as red cell viability is maintained and plasma proteins remain functional. This anticoagulant may be purchased from a commercial veterinary blood bank in multi-use vials or withdrawn from a blood bag port using a syringe (Kohn and Weingart, 2012).

Closed Systems

Blood collection systems used for canine blood collection are not suitable for collection of feline blood since the volume of anticoagulant in the blood collection bag is intended for a 450 ml blood draw. Although the amount of anticoagulant could be reduced in order to accommodate a smaller blood draw, the integrally attached 16-gauge collection needle is too large for the feline jugular vein used to collect blood. For these reasons, blood bags used for the collection of canine blood are not used for cats.

A specialized blood collection system for cats is available through Animal Blood Resources (Figure 2.7). The system contains an integrally attached 19 gauge needle, and two systems are available that allow blood to be collected via syringe or with the use of a vacuum chamber. CPDA-1 is the preferred anticoagulant as this allows for maximum refrigerated shelf life.

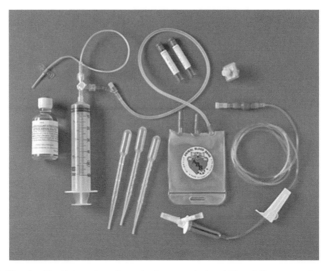

Figure 2.7 Blood collection system for cats. Source: Animal Blood Resources International. Reproduced with permission.

References and Further Reading

American Association of Blood Banks (2013). Circular of information for the use of human blood and blood components. Available at: www.aabb.org/tm/coi/Documents/coi1113.pdf

Animal Blood Resources International (ABRI). Available at: www.abrint.net

Arteaga J. (2014) Technology of a high performance blood bank refrigerator. Available at: www.mlo-online.com/technology-of-a-high-performance-blood-bank-refrigerator.php

Day MJ. (2012) Feline blood groups and blood typing. In: *BSAVA Manual of Canine and Feline Haematology and Transfusion Medicine*, 2nd edn. Day MJ, Kohn B, eds., pp. 285–288. Gloucester: British Small Animal Veterinary Association.

ECRI Institute (2012) Hospital medical equipment, refrigerator blood bank. Available at: www.who.int/medical_devices/innovation/hospt_equip_28.pdf

Feldman BF, Sink CA. (2006) Collection, processing, storage, and shipment. In: *Practical Transfusion Medicine for the Small Animal Practitioner*, pp. 15–43. Jackson, WY: Teton NewMedia.

Fenwal website. Available at: www.fenwalinc.com

Ferreira RF, Gopegui RR, Araujo MM, de Matos AJ. (2014) Effects of repeated blood donations on iron status and hematologic variables of canine blood donors. *J Am Vet Med Assoc* 244(11): 1298–1303.

Gibson G. (2007) Transfusion medicine. In: *BSAVA Manual of Canine and Feline Emergency and Critical Care*, 2nd edn. King LG, Boag A, eds., pp. 215–227. Gloucester: British Small Animal Veterinary Association.

Gibson G, Abrams-Ogg A. (2012) Canine transfusion medicine. In: *BSAVA Manual of Canine and Feline Haematology and Transfusion Medicine*, 2nd edn. Day MJ, Kohn B, eds., pp. 289–307. Gloucester: British Small Animal Veterinary Association.

JMS website. Available at: www.jmss.com.sg/product_portfolio/equipment_plasma_extractor.htm

Kilos MB, Graham LF, Lee J. (2010) Comparison of two aesthetic protocols for feline blood donation. *Vet Anaesth Analg* (37): 230–239.

Kohn B, Weingart C. (2012) Feline transfusion medicine. In: *BSAVA Manual of Canine and Feline Haematology and Transfusion Medicine*, 2nd edn. Day MJ, Kohn B, eds., pp. 309–318. Gloucester: British Small Animal Veterinary Association.

Terumo website. Available at: www.terumomedical.com

Waldrop KJ. (1995) Selection of anticoagulant-preservatives for canine and feline blood storage. *Vet Clin North Am Small Animal Practice* 25(6): 1323–1332.

Yagi K. (2016) Transfusion medicine. In: *Small Animal Emergency and Critical Care for Veterinary Technicians*, 3rd edn. Battaglia AM, Steele AM., eds., pp. 78–105. Philadelphia, PA: Saunders.

Chapter 3 Blood Products Overview

Introduction

Using closed blood collection systems, veterinary blood banks routinely separate units of whole blood into components, maximizing blood utilization and facilitating the treatment of multiple patients from a single unit of blood. The most commonly used blood components in veterinary medicine will be described.

Blood Components

Whole Blood and Red Cells
Fresh Whole Blood

Fresh whole blood provides blood volume expansion and increased oxygen-carrying capacity to the recipient. It also delivers viable platelets and coagulation factors. It is often used for actively bleeding patients with acute blood volume loss greater than 25%.

A unit of whole blood is called fresh whole blood for 24 hours after phlebotomy. Fresh whole blood contains all blood elements: red cells, platelets, clotting factors, and plasma proteins, and is stored at 1–6°C. ACD, CPD, CP2D, and CPDA-1 are suitable anticoagulant–preservatives but red cell additives are not mixed with whole blood.

Because of its limited vitality, fresh whole blood is generally not available unless it is drawn immediately prior to its need. Since obtaining a blood donor on an emergency basis is not usually practical, it may not be feasible to routinely transfuse fresh whole blood. Instead, fresh whole blood is generally used for component preparation.

Practical Transfusion Medicine for the Small Animal Practitioner, Second Edition. Carolyn A. Sink.
© 2017 John Wiley & Sons, Inc. Published 2017 by John Wiley & Sons, Inc.
Companion website: www.wiley.com/go/sink/transfusion

Whole Blood or Stored Whole Blood

Whole blood provides for volume expansion, increased oxygen-carrying capacity, protein source, and stable coagulation factors. Once fresh whole blood is stored at 1–6°C for longer than 24 hours, it is classified as whole blood or stored whole blood. Whole blood contains red cells and plasma proteins, but platelets and coagulation factors are diminished. Stable coagulation factors II, VII, IX, X, and fibrinogen are preserved. The anticoagulant–preservatives ACD, CPD, and CP2DA maintain this product for 21 days. The use of CPDA-1 maintains whole blood for 35 days.

Red cell additives are not mixed with whole blood. Stored whole blood is an option for extending the use of a unit of fresh whole blood once the 24-hour shelf life is exceeded.

Short Draw

Most commercially available blood bags are intended for a 450 ml + 45 ml blood volume. These bags contain 63 ml of anticoagulant–preservative for a final blood-to-anticoagulant ratio of 1:10.

If 300–404 ml of blood is drawn into a bag intended for a 450 ml blood draw, components should not be made from this unit and the unit should be maintained as whole blood. It can be used for transfusion, but it should be labeled as a low-volume unit. These under-filled units can cause citrate intoxication if transfused.

If a blood collection of less than 300 ml of blood is needed, the amount of anticoagulant–preservative may be aseptically reduced prior to blood collection (Table 3.1).

Red Blood Cells

Also called packed cells, red blood cells assist in restoring oxygen-carrying capacity to the recipient with less expansion of blood volume in comparison to whole blood. Red blood cells are used to treat anemia in normovolemic patients or pharmacologically untreatable anemia.

Red blood cells are prepared from a unit of fresh whole blood or whole blood. To prepare this product, plasma is extracted from the unit of whole blood and the cells remaining in the bag are called red cells (or packed cells). This process

Table 3.1 Decreasing the amount of anticoagulant-preservative in a closed blood collection system

Amount of anticoagulant–preservative needed in ml	= (ml of blood to be drawn/100) × 14 ml
Amount of anticoagulant–preservative to remove from the primary blood bag	= 63 ml – Amount of anticoagulant-preservative needed in ml*

* This calculation is valid only for anticoagulant-preservatives on which the ratio of anticoagulant to blood is 1.4:10 (i.e., CPD or CPDA-1).

Table 3.2 Red cell blood products

Product	Contains
Fresh whole blood	All blood elements: red cells, platelets, clotting factors
Whole blood, stored whole blood	Red cells, plasma proteins, stable coagulation factors
Red blood cells, packed cells	Red cells

is best expedited by centrifugation but the red cells may be allowed to settle to the bottom of an undisturbed unit of whole blood. ACD, CPD, and CP2D provide a shelf life of 21 days at 1–6°C. CPDA-1 provides for a shelf life of 35 days. Packed cells can be prepared from whole blood at any time before the expiration date.

Red cell additives will extend the life of a unit of red cells to 42 days when stored at 1–6°C. Red blood cell additives must be mixed with red cells within 72 hours of phlebotomy.

Red blood cells may contain approximately 20–100 ml of residual plasma. Packed cells prepared with additive solutions are the most commonly used red cell product and have limited residual plasma.

A summary of blood products containing red cells can be found in Table 3.2.

Plasma Products
Fresh Frozen Plasma

Fresh frozen plasma (FFP) contains all the coagulation factors including labile Factors V, VIII, and von Willebrand factor (VWF). It is a source of plasma proteins and is a volume expander. FFP is used for treatment of patients with inadequate clotting factors for any reason. It is also used for vitamin K deficiency or antagonism, disseminated intravascular coagulation, severe liver disease and can be used prophylactically in patients with known coagulopathies. FFP used in conjunction with red blood cells provides most of the benefits of fresh whole blood.

FFP is prepared from a unit of fresh whole blood. The plasma is separated from the red cells by centrifugation and removed. It is then completely frozen at −18°C or lower. Complete freezing of the plasma must occur within 8 hours of phlebotomy if the anticoagulant–preservative is CPD, CP2D, or CPDA-1. If ACD is used, separation and freezing must occur within 6 hours of phlebotomy. Once frozen, the product has a shelf life of 1 year from the original phlebotomy date.

Plasma or Stored Frozen Plasma

Plasma is used to treat stable clotting factor deficiencies. This product contains vitamin K-dependent factors, albumin, and immunoglobulins. It may be used as a volume expander in warfarin/coumarin toxicity or canine parvovirus.

This product is derived from extending the shelf life of a unit of FFP. When a unit of FFP is stored at −18°C for longer than one year, it can be relabeled as plasma or stored frozen plasma. This is done to reflect the loss of clotting factors that occurs during the one-year storage. Plasma has a shelf life of 5 years from the original phlebotomy date. Plasma not separated from red blood cells within 6–8 hours after phlebotomy is labeled plasma (not FFP).

Cryoprecipitated Anti-hemophilic Factor

Cryoprecipitated anti-hemophilic factor (cryoprecipitate, cryo, or AHF) is a rich source of VWF, Factor VIII, fibrinogen, Factor XIII, and fibronectin. It is useful in the treatment of von Willebrand disease, hemophilia A, hypofibrinogenemia, disseminated intravascular coagulation, and septicemia.

The use of desmopressin in blood donors at 0.6 μg/kg body weight, diluted in 15 ml of physiological saline, administered by slow injection 30–60 minutes prior to blood donation may increase the amount of VWF in the donor plasma and increase the yield of cryoprecipitate (Johnstone, 1999).

Cryoprecipitate is made from a unit of FFP. FFP contains high molecular weight plasma proteins that precipitate in a cold environment. When a unit of FFP is thawed at 1–6°C, the resulting precipitate is cryoprecipitated AHF. After approximately 90% of the plasma is removed, cryoprecipitated AHF is refrozen and maintained at −18°C or lower; it has a shelf life of one year from the original phlebotomy date.

Cryoprecipitate-poor Plasma

Cryoprecipitate-poor plasma (cryo-poor, plasma cryoprecipitate reduced, CPP) contains very low amounts of fibrinogen, fibronectin, Factors XI, XIII, VII, and VWF. It contains no Factor V. Cryo-poor plasma contains the vitamin K-dependent factors albumin and globulins. It is suitable for treatment of canine parvovirus or coumarin/warfarin toxicity.

Cryo-poor plasma is the residual plasma left from making cryoprecipitated anti-hemophilic factor. When maintained at −18°C or lower it has a shelf life of one year from the original phlebotomy date.

Platelets

Platelets stop hemorrhage as they are the first cellular element of the peripheral blood to react when blood vessels are damaged. Platelet concentrates or platelet-rich plasma are prepared immediately after blood collection using differential centrifugation. The freshly collected unit of blood should not be refrigerated prior to blood processing and should be maintained between 22 and 25°C.

Platelet-rich plasma is separated from fresh whole blood using a light spin (2000 *g* for 3 minutes). Platelet concentrates are separated from platelet-rich plasma using a hard spin (5000 *g* for 5 minutes.) The residual plasma can be stored as FFP or plasma (as appropriate).

Platelets are viable for at least 5 days from the phlebotomy date when stored between 22 and 25°C. In order to prevent platelet aggregation and to provide adequate oxygen and carbon dioxide exchange, platelet products should undergo

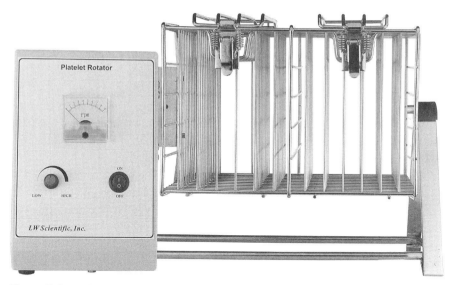

Figure 3.1 Two-basket platelet rotator. Source: LW Scientific. Reproduced with permission.

a rest period of up to 1 hour; the product should be left label side down at 22–25°C during the rest period (Moroff *et al.*, 2006) and then stored with gentle, continuous agitation. Platelet rotators are widely used in blood banks that store platelets (Figure 3.1).

Further Processing
Leukocyte Reduction
Donor leukocytes can cause adverse reactions in the recipient during transfusion. Leukocyte-reduced blood products have been shown to eliminate or attenuate adverse response to transfusion. Removal of white blood cells from a blood component can be achieved by in-process collection or filtration: pre-storage, after varying periods of storage, or during blood administration. Leukocyte reduction will decrease the cellular content and volume of blood (primarily leukocytes and platelets) according to characteristics of the filter system used. Leukocyte reduction filters variably remove other cellular elements in addition to white cells.

Irradiated Blood Components
In human medicine, blood and blood components may be irradiated prior to transfusion to prevent the proliferation of certain types of T lymphocytes that can inhibit the immune response and cause graft-versus-host disease (American Association of Blood Banks, 2013).

Irradiation is performed using method-validated self-contained blood irradiators or hospital radiation therapy machines.

Lyophilized Blood Components

Lyophilized components, including platelets and cryoprecipitate, are gaining popularity in veterinary medicine. These products offer increased concentration, decreased volumes, and longer storage shelf life (Hux and Martin, 2012), although production of these components is limited to specialized laboratories.

References and Further Reading

American Association of Blood Banks (2013) Circular of information for the use of human blood and blood components. Available at: www.aabb.org/tm/coi/Documents/coi1113.pdf

Davenport M. (2007) Transfusion medicine. In: *Henry's Clinical Diagnosis and Management by Laboratory Methods*, 21st edn. McPherson RA, Pincus MR, eds., pp. 669–684. Philadelphia, PA: WB Saunders.

Hux BD, Martin LG. (2012) Platelet transfusions: treatment options for hemorrhage secondary to thrombocytopenia. *J Vet Emerg Crit Care* 22(1): 73–80.

Johnstone IB. (1999) Desmopressin enhances the binding of plasma von Willebrand factor to collagen in plasmas from normal dogs and dogs with type I von Willebrand's disease. *Can Vet J* 40(9): 645–648.

Kikuyo Notomi M, Ruiz de Gopegui R, Escodro PB. (2015) Haematologic effects of leukoreduction on canine whole blood post-filtration and post-storage. *Comp Clin Pathol* 25(1): 145–149.

McMichael MA, Smith SA, Galligan A, Swanson KS, Fan TM. (2010) Effect of leukoreduction on transfusion-induced inflammation in dogs. *J Vet Intern Med* 24: 1131–1137.

Moroff G, Kline L, Dabay M, Hunter S, Johnson A, McNeil D, Nixon J, Sawyer S, Taylor H, Whitley P, Wahab F, Murphy S. (2006) Reevaluation of the resting time period when preparing whole blood-derived platelet concentrates with the platelet-rich plasma method. *Transfusion* 46(4): 572–577.

Rajesh CA, Wander GS, Pankaj G. (2011) Blood component therapy: Which, when and how much. *J Anaesthesiol Clin Pharmacol* 27(2): 278–284.

Chapter 4 Clinical Considerations in Transfusion Practice

Introduction

Modern transfusion therapy is based upon the use of components to treat specific defects with concentrates of the deficient blood constituent. As blood transfusions are associated with certain risks, transfusion therapy should only be initiated when laboratory pre-transfusion testing is complete and the expected benefits of the transfusion outweigh the potential risks.

Laboratory Evaluation for Pre-transfusion Testing

Blood Typing

Blood types are species specific and the relevance of a blood type is related to its antigenicity. Ideally, dogs and cats should be blood typed prior to transfusion in an effort to minimize adverse reaction to transfusion, either by immediate hemolysis of infused cells or by alloantibody response due to exposure to a foreign red cell antigen.

Canine

The most significant blood group in dogs is DEA 1.1. DEA 1.1-positive connotes that DEA 1.1 antigen is present on the red cells, a trait which DEA 1.1-negative dogs lack. Point-of-care DEA 1.1 blood typing assays are available and discussed in Chapter 6.

In dogs, universal blood type means that the donor is negative for all DEA types (except DEA 4). The clinical significance of DEA 3, 5, and 7 is variable and typing for these antigens is available through specialized laboratories. This extended blood typing is yet to be designed for clinical use, likely because of the low risk of significant reaction to DEA 3, 5, or 7 during the first transfusion (see Table 1.7).

Practical Transfusion Medicine for the Small Animal Practitioner, Second Edition. Carolyn A. Sink.
© 2017 John Wiley & Sons, Inc. Published 2017 by John Wiley & Sons, Inc.
Companion website: www.wiley.com/go/sink/transfusion

Feline

Cats should always be blood typed prior to transfusion. The feline AB blood group consists of three blood types: A, B, and AB. While 96–99% of domestic shorthair cats are type A, certain breeds have increased prevalence of type B (see Table 1.9). Type AB is extremely rare and any AB blood type result should be verified by repeat laboratory analysis. Point-of-care blood typing assays are available, as discussed in Chapter 6.

Type A cats possess A antigen on the red cell surface, type B cats possess B, and AB cats possess both. In the plasma, type A cats have generally weak anti-B antibodies and type AB cats have no alloantibodies (related to A or B antigens). Type B cats possess strong anti-A antibodies.

The Crossmatch

The major and minor crossmatches are performed to assist in providing compatible red cell products and possibly alleviating adverse reactions to transfusion. The major crossmatch is performed to detect antibodies in the recipient's plasma that may agglutinate or lyse the donor's erythrocytes. Conversely, the minor crossmatch detects antibodies in donor plasma directed against recipient erythrocytes. Most often, a positive minor crossmatch is relevant only if large amounts of plasma are being administered to the patient or if whole blood will be used.

A crossmatch should always be performed when:

- the transfusion status of the patient is not known;
- 4 days or more following a red cell transfusion (whole blood or red blood cells);
- the patient has a history of transfusion reaction(s).

Canine

A DEA 1.1-positive dog can receive either DEA 1.1-positive or -negative red cells, while DEA 1.1-negative dogs should only receive DEA 1.1-negative cells. For first time transfusion, a crossmatch is not required and type-specific blood can be dispensed. As alloantibodies can be produced within 4 days of exposure, the crossmatch should be performed for subsequent transfusions 4 days later than the first.

Feline

Type B cats have very strong anti-A antibodies that can cause serious, even fatal, hemolytic transfusion reactions when as little as 1 ml of type A blood is transfused to a type B cat. For this reason, type-specific red cells should be dispensed for the first transfusion. Subsequent transfusions require crossmatching as outlined above.

While crossmatching is not necessary for plasma products, it is absolutely necessary to transfuse AB compatible plasma to cats.

A summary of red cell selection guidelines is given in Table 4.1.

Table 4.1 Guidelines for selecting and dispensing red blood cells (RBC)

Canine	
Based on DEA 1.1 blood type results as follows:	
Recipient 1.1-negative	Use RBC that are 1.1-negative
Recipient 1.1-positive	Use RBC that are 1.1-positive
If type-specific RBC are not available:	
Recipient 1.1-negative	Use universal RBC
If neither 1.1-negative nor universal RBC are available	Use 1.1-positive RBC
Recipient 1.1-positive	Use 1.1-negative red cells
If neither 1.1-positive nor 1.1-negative RBC are available	Use universal RBC
Feline	
Based on AB blood type as follows:	
Recipient type A	Use type A RBC
Recipient type B (rare)	Use type B RBC
Recipient type AB (rare)	Use type A RBC

Source: Virginia Tech Animal Laboratory Services (2015).

Considerations for Transfusion

Limited Resource

The most cogent argument supporting component therapy is that blood is a precious resource considering its therapeutic potential and the logistics and costs required in obtaining and delivering blood products. Separation of whole blood into components permits a single donation to meet the individual needs of several patients.

Kinetic

Following hemorrhage, homeostatic mechanisms restore the various blood constituents at differing rates, depending on the capacity for synthesis, endogenous consumption, degradation, and distribution in various physiologic compartments. The half-inactivation time of canine and feline red cells is in terms of months, whereas the half-life of albumin is just 3–4 days. Surgical blood loss may require restoration of blood cells. Albumin may not be required, as it is restored within several days. Another consideration is tolerance. Loss of 50% of blood volume can be fatal unless rapidly corrected.

Adverse Effects

Other rationale for supporting the use of blood components include the myriad of possible side effects that can result from transfusion of unnecessary blood constituents. Any transfusion reaction means that the transfusion is not performing the intended job and, importantly, has burdened a patient already burdened by the physiologic state requiring transfusion. Sensitization to blood cells can result in refractory results in subsequent transfusions. Transfusion of multiple units of whole blood sequentially in order to achieve a certain hematocrit may also produce pulmonary edema due to volume overload.

The Decision to Transfuse

All transfusion therapy can produce only transient improvement in the patient's condition. Unless the patient is able to produce the deficit component endogenously, more transfusions will be necessary. Furthermore, transfusions dampen the physiologic response to deficiency of a blood constituent. For example, if the patient has a low red cell mass, tissue hypoxia results in increased erythropoietin production and the marrow responds with reticulocytosis. Red cell transfusion in this patient will result in diminished and delayed reticulocyte response. See Table 4.2 for additional transfusion considerations.

Transfusion Considerations for Blood Components
Red-cell-containing components are indicated for treatment of symptomatic or critical deficit of oxygen-carrying capacity.

Whole blood and red cell components increase the recipient's oxygen-carrying capacity by increasing the mass of circulating red cells. Plasma components contain coagulation factors and plasma proteins; identification of the patient's hemostatic abnormality is necessary for component selection and therapy (see Table 4.2).

Transfusion to Increase Oxygen Transport
There is no set hemoglobin or hematocrit concentration below which a patient needs red cells. Patients and patient care dictate when red cells are required. A patient who has lost one third of their red cell mass acutely will require increase oxygen-carrying capacity. Patients with chronic processes may have dramatically low hematocrits and, if not stressed, may not require additional oxygen-carrying capacity. However, in general terms, in both the dog and the cat, administering red cells to meet oxygen transport needs should be considered when hemoglobin concentration is below 7 g/dl (hematocrit of 21%). When considering transfusion in specific patients, the clinician should consider age, etiology and duration of anemia, presence of coexisting cardiac, pulmonary, or vascular conditions, and hemodynamic stability.

Table 4.2 Considerations prior to transfusion

Is the blood transfusion really necessary?
What is this patient's particular need?
Does the prospective benefit justify the risks of transfusion?
What blood component will effectively meet this special need at the lowest cost?
After transfusion: Did the transfusion result in the anticipated benefit for the patient?

Products that Increase Oxygen Transport

Whole blood can be used during acute massive blood loss exceeding 20% of blood volume (approximate blood volume is 90 ml/kg – canine, 70 ml/kg – feline) or coagulopathy with massive blood loss. The hematocrit will increase over the baseline value immediately after transfusion and increases further within 24 hours with volume redistribution.

The hematocrit of a unit of red cells (packed cells) will approximate 70–80% with a volume between 225 and 350 ml. Red cells are often mixed with sterile saline or with an additive solution to increase viscosity. Additive solutions may be mixed with the red cells remaining after removal of nearly all of the plasma; the typical hematocrit is 55–65% and the volume is approximately 300–400 ml. Table 4.3 outlines red cell component selection.

Transfusion to Correct Coagulopathy or Plasma Proteins Deficiency

Constituents of plasma blood components include coagulation factors, plasma proteins, and/or platelets. Selection of the appropriate blood component is dependent on correct diagnosis of the hemostatic event (Table 4.4). In addition

Table 4.3 Red cell component selection guidelines

Product name	Contains	Indication	Comments
Fresh whole blood	Red cells Plasma proteins Coagulation factors Platelets	Severe hemorrhage due to thrombocytopenia	Use immediately. Refrigeration interferes with platelet function
Stored whole blood	Red cells Plasma proteins Coagulation factors	Anemia	Individual component therapy better
Red blood cells	Red cells	Anemia	Oxygen-carrying benefit but less volume than whole blood

Table 4.4 Plasma component selection guidelines

Product name	Contains	Indication	Comments
Fresh frozen plasma	Coagulation factors Plasma Albumin	Factor deficiencies	Thaw for 30 minutes maximum at 37 °C
Cryoprecipitate	Factor VIII Von Willebrand factor Fibrinogen Fibronectin	Factor VIII deficiency Von Willebrand disease Hypofibrinogenemia	Thaw for 15 minutes maximum at 37 °C
Platelet-rich plasma or platelet concentrate	Platelets Plasma	Thrombocytopenia	Usually a special request product

to the products listed in Table 4.4, some commercial veterinary blood banks also produce lyophilized cryoprecipitate, lyophilized albumin, and frozen platelet concentrates (leukoreduced) for dogs; these products have the benefit of extended shelf life.

Alternatives to Blood and Blood Products

Since no synthetic product fulfills all the attributes of blood, substitute products, delineated by the attribute in which they fulfill, are described below.

Hemoglobin-based Oxygen-carrying Solutions

Requirements and clinical indications for red cell substitute are found in Table 4.5. Hemoglobin-based oxygen-carrying solutions (HBOCS) are used to increase the oxygen content of blood and improve oxygen delivery to tissues. Hemoglobin is carried in the plasma and increases the efficiency of offloading oxygen from blood cells to tissues by facilitating diffusion of oxygen through the plasma. HBOCS have a long shelf life (3 years at room temperature) and are useful immediately. These solutions are polymerized stroma-free hemoglobin, which are virtually free of red cell membranes and as such are minimally immunogenic. These solutions deliver and release oxygen for 18–24 hours.

Because of the intense red color of HBOCS, some laboratory assays are affected and laboratory results vary by the test methodology that is employed. Additionally, administration of these solutions turns mucous membranes yellow to red to brown for at least several days.

At the time of writing this chapter, Oxyglobin (HbO$_2$ Therapeutics, Souderton, PA, USA), remains a registered HBOC pharmaceutical, available in Europe and Canada. Anticipated release date for the United States market is mid 2017 (Zafiris Zafireli, 2016, personal communication).

Table 4.5 Red cell substitutes

Requirements:	It must work
	Have a long shelf life
	Be minimally immunogenic
	Be pathogen and endotoxin free
	Be readily available at a reasonable cost
	Must deliver and release oxygen to tissues under clinical conditions
Clinical indications:	Acute anemia
	Acute blood loss
	Preoperative therapy
	Intraoperative replacement

Plasma Substitutes

Hetastarch is a synthetic polymer (waxy starch amylopectin) produced by DuPont Pharmaceuticals under the name Hespan®. It is 6% hetastarch in normal saline which is almost iso-osmotic (310 mOsm/L). Hespan has a shelf life of 12 months.

Albumin is indicated for hypoalbuminemia or the treatment of hypovolemic shock. Administration of the product provides temporary replacement of albumin and is not intended as long-term therapy for hypoalbuminemia or clinical shock. Lyophilized canine albumin has a shelf life of 36 months, is stored at 2–6 °C and has a 24-hour expiration date once reconstituted.

Compatible IV Solutions

A 0.9% sodium chloride injection may be used to facilitate infusion of blood products. No medications or any other solution should be added to blood products unless the product is approved by the US Food and Drug Administration or there is adequate documentation that the product is safe for use with blood products.

Various intravenous solutions interfere with blood transfusion. Lactated Ringer's solution contains enough calcium to overcome chelating agents in anticoagulant–preservative additive systems, which results in clot formation in the infusion line. Five per cent dextrose in water causes red cells to clump in the in the infusion line, causing red cells to swell and hemolyze.

Preparation of Blood Products for Transfusion

Warming red cell products can lead to hemolysis of the red cells and creates a favorable environment for proliferation of microbial contaminants (if present). Stored red cell products need not be warmed prior to use unless the animal is hypothermic or receiving large volumes of blood (rapidly), or if the animal is of very small size or a neonate. If warming of the red cell product is absolutely necessary, the unit of blood should be placed in a zip closure bag and warmed in a circulating water bath. The water bath should be closely monitored or controlled so that the temperature does not exceed 37 °C. Do not microwave the product.

Frozen plasma products must be thawed prior to transfusion. Product can be placed in a zip closure bag and warmed in a circulating water bath that is closely monitored or controlled so that the temperature does not exceed 37 °C. A dry thawing and warming device is also available (Genesis™ Plasmatherm) (Figure 4.1). Frozen products should not be thawed using conventional microwave.

Stored blood components should be visually inspected daily and immediately prior to use. Although visual inspection cannot always detect contamination

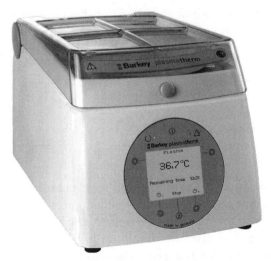

Figure 4.1 Genesis™ Plasmatherm. Source: GenesisBPS. Reproduced with permission.

Table 4.6 Potential reasons to quarantine or discard stored red cell products

Plasma/supernatant is murky, purple, brown or red
The red cell mass has changed color (bright red, purple, etc.)
A zone of hemolysis or green sheen is observed just above the red cell mass
Clots are visible
Red cells in the segments are lighter than those in the bag

or deleterious conditions, blood products that appear abnormal should not be used. See Table 4.6 for conditions of suspected contamination for red cell products.

Visual inspection for stored frozen plasma products should include a method to detect thawing and refreezing during storage, as product efficacy could be compromised. The unit should not be used if the bag or tubing is torn or cracked. Unusual turbidity in thawed components is a reason to discard.

Stored platelet products should be inspected for excessive aggregates.

Initiating Blood Administration

Prior to transfusion, identification of the transfusion component and the intended recipient should be verified.

Both the appearance of the blood component and the expiration date should be checked to make sure the unit is suitable for transfusion; likewise, blood group and/or compatibility testing (if performed) should be confirmed. Any discrepancy should be resolved prior to beginning the transfusion.

Baseline parameters including attitude, patient temperature, pulse rate, mucous membrane color, respiratory rate and character, and capillary refill time, packed cell volume (PCV), total protein, and plasma color should be documented.

The above parameters should be monitored every 15–30 minutes during transfusion and periodically thereafter (1, 12, and 24 hours).

Blood Administration

Infusion Sets

Blood administration sets are used for the infusion of blood products. The use of a blood administration set assists in preventing potentially dangerous artifacts from being infused to the recipient. Sets contain a filter that serves to retain clots and other microaggregate particles that form in stored blood. The size of the particle retained by the filter is directly related to the size of the filter.

Blood administration sets should be used with all blood components, including platelet concentrates. Manufacturer's instructions should be followed to avoid rendering the blood product ineffective (see Table 4.5). For example, using an inappropriate administration set for the infusion of platelet products could cause platelets to be retained within the infusion set, defeating the purpose of the transfusion.

There are a variety of configurations of infusion sets commercially available.

Gravity Drip

Standard blood administration sets contain a filter with a pore size of 170–260 μm. The set should be primed according to the manufacturer's directions with blood or blood-compatible fluid. For optimal flow rate, the filter should be fully wet and the drip chamber should be no more than half full during transfusion. Standard sets are typically used to transfuse whole blood, red cells, and plasma products. As the name implies, this set is attached to the blood product and the blood product is infused by gravity drip.

Syringe Push

Syringe push sets may be used for component infusion or in the transfusion of products with a volume of less than 100 ml. This blood administration set uses the smallest priming volume of all sets. Some sets have a smaller drip chamber and shorter tubing length than gravity infusion sets. This is helpful in the transfusion of small volume products. The Hemo-Nate® Microaggregate Blood Filtration System (Utah Medical) syringe push sets contain an 18 μm in-line filter that is extremely small and it may go unnoticed. The filter is not indicated as an antibacterial or antimicrobial filter.

Blood products may be transfused in one of two ways using this infusion set. The set may be attached to a blood bag, the product drawn into the attached

Table 4.7 Blood administration rates after loading dose*

Product	Canine	Feline
Whole blood	20 ml/kg	5–10 ml/kg per hour
Red cells	10–12 ml/kg	10–20 ml/kg
FFP	6–20 ml/kg per hour	6–20 ml/kg per hour
Cryo	2–5 ml/kg over 2 hours	

* The recommendations, dosages and rates on this chart are presented as a guideline and are not a substitute for the veterinarian's clinical evaluation of an individual patient's condition.
Source: Data from Animal Blood Resources International (www.abrint.net).

syringe and pushed into the recipient. Alternately, this set may be attached directly to a syringe of blood for immediate transfusion. This may be useful for smaller transfusion volumes, as in the transfusion of feline whole blood.

Blood Administration Rates

Blood administration rates are shown in Table 4.7. In general, for red cells or FFP in dogs, the average volume for infusion is 6–12 ml/kg. The transfusion is initiated at a slow infusion rate: 0.25–1.0 ml/kg per hour for the first 20 minutes for dogs, 1–3 ml over 5 minutes for cats. The patient should be monitored for signs of incompatibility. After that, the infusion rate is dependent on cardiovascular status of the recipient. The rate can be increased so that the remaining product is infused within 4 hours.

References and Further Reading

Adamik KN, Yozova ID, Regenscheit N. (2015) Controversies in the use of hydroxyethyl starch solutions in small animal emergency and critical care. *J Vet Emerg Crit Care* 25(1): 20–47.

Animal Blood Resources International (ABRI). Available at: www.abrint.net

Brown D, Vap L. (2012) Principles of blood transfusion and crossmatching. In: *Veterinary Hematology and Clinical Chemistry*, 2nd edn., Thrall MA, Weiser G, Allison RW, Campbell TW, eds., pp. 205–222. Ames, IA: John Wiley & Sons.

Merck Veterinary Manual (2013) Blood substitutes: hemoglobin-based oxygen carrier solution. Available at: www.merckvetmanual.com/mvm/circulatory_system/blood_groups_and_blood_transfusions/blood_substitutes_hemoglobin-based_oxygen_carrier_solutions.html

Utah Medical. Available at: www.utahmed.com/hemonate.htm

Virginia Tech Animal Laboratory Services (2015) Blood Bank Procedure Manual (unpublished). Virginia Maryland College of Veterinary Medicine.

Yagi K. (2016) Transfusion medicine. In: *Small Animal Emergency and Critical Care for Veterinary Technicians*, 3rd edn. Battaglia AM, Steele AM, eds., pp. 78–103. Philadelphia, PA: Saunders.

Yaxley PE, Beal MW, Jutkowitz LA, Hauptman JG, Brooks MB, Hale AS. (2010) comparative stability of canine and feline hemostatic proteins in freeze-that-cycled fresh frozen plasma. *J Vet Emerg Crit Care* 20(5): 472–478.

Chapter 5 Adverse Effects of Blood Transfusion

Introduction

The basic principle in transfusion therapy is the same as in all medical approaches: "primum non nocere" – first, do no harm. While blood transfusions are fairly common and considered to be safe, complications – collectively known as transfusion reactions – occur. Transfusion reactions can develop during the transfusion or weeks or months after the transfusion. Safe transfusion practices include the appropriated pre-transfusion testing for donors and recipients, careful observation of the recipient's clinical signs during transfusion and appropriate evaluation of any adverse effect from transfusion. This chapter provides a general outline of the clinical signs and the associated physiologic mechanisms of transfusion reactions.

Signs of Transfusion Reactions

Febrile or allergic reactions may occur in the same manner as severe hemolytic reaction. For this reason, any change in the patient's condition during blood infusion should be considered a possible sign of adverse reaction and should be evaluated.

If a transfusion reaction is suspected the following steps are essential:

- Stop the transfusion.
- Keep intravenous access patent for treatment if necessary.
- Notify the responsible clinician to evaluate the patient.

Acute Hemolytic Transfusion Reactions

Acute hemolytic transfusion reactions occur within 24 hours of a red cell transfusion. Primarily mediated by immunoglobulin G (IgG), they are antigen–antibody, type 2 hypersensitivity reactions and result in an abrupt hemolytic transfusion reaction with intravascular hemolysis. These reactions are severe, but rare,

---

Practical Transfusion Medicine for the Small Animal Practitioner, Second Edition. Carolyn A. Sink.
© 2017 John Wiley & Sons, Inc. Published 2017 by John Wiley & Sons, Inc.
Companion website: www.wiley.com/go/sink/transfusion

and are due to incompatible blood or previously sensitized alloantibody-mediated incompatibility (i.e., the recipient either has a naturally occurring alloantibody to the donor's red blood cells or the recipient has been sensitized through a previous transfusion and has pre-formed antibodies that react and lyse infused cells).

In cats, because of naturally occurring alloantibodies, type A blood infused to a type B recipient can be fatal. Since dogs lack clinically significant red cell alloantibodies, acute hemolytic transfusion reactions are primarily caused by sensitization from a previous blood transfusion (or possibly through pregnancy).

Possible clinical signs of an acute immune-mediated hemolytic transfusion reaction include hemoglobinemia, hemoglobinuria, fever, tachycardia, dyspnea, and vomiting.

Prevention of this type of transfusion reaction includes pre-transfusion blood type and crossmatch (Weinstein, 2010).

Delayed Hemolytic Transfusion Reactions

Delayed hemolytic transfusion reactions occur more than 24 hours after transfusion, with onset varying from 2 to 21 days. These reactions are often the result of an amnestic response to a red cell antigen that the recipient lacks (i.e., the recipient has previously produced the reactive alloantibody but it was at low concentration before transfusion). This type of reaction can also be due to primary alloimmunization to a red cell antigen.

A delayed hemolytic transfusion reaction should be suspected if the patient's PCV decreases more rapidly than expected post transfusion. Clinical signs of a delayed hemolytic transfusion reaction include hyperbilirubinemia, bilirubinuria, jaundice, anorexia, and fever (often unnoticed).

Prevention of this type of transfusion reaction includes pre-transfusion blood type and crossmatch.

Non-hemolytic Transfusion Reactions: Allergic and Febrile

These are the most common types of transfusion reaction. Allergic reactions are often associated with transfusion of plasma products that contain a substance to which the recipient has been sensitized. Signs of an allergic reaction typically begin within 15 minutes of infusion and include urticarial, pruritus, and erythema; additional signs include nausea, vomiting, or diarrhea. Treatment includes decreasing the infusion rate and administration of an antihistamine.

Febrile, non-hemolytic transfusion reactions are associated with recipient alloantibodies that react with antigens present on donor lymphocytes, granulocytes, or platelets. These are characterized by an increase in patient temperature

Table 5.1 Uncommon immunologic transfusion reactions

Reaction	Cause
Anaphylaxis secondary to IgA deficiency	Recipient anti-IgA antibodies react to IgA in donor plasma
Veterinary acute lung injury (VetALI)	Dyspnea, hypoxia, non-cardiogenic pulmonary edema
Post-transfusion purpura	Recipient produces anti-platelet antibodies
Transfusion-associated graft-vs-host disease	Transfusion-associated graft-vs-host disease

Source: Thomovsky and Bach (2014), Weinstein (2010).

Table 5.2 Non-immunologic transfusion reactions

Reaction	Prevention
Infectious disease	Appropriate donor screening
Sepsis due to transfusion	Strict adherence to processing and infusion procedures Infuse product within 4 hours
Citrate toxicity	Counteract with intravenous calcium as appropriate
Circulatory overload	Management of fluid infusion, treat with diuretics as appropriate

during or within 4 hours of infusion. Additional clinical signs include vomiting and tremors. Leukoreduction of red cell components has potential for minimizing this type of transfusion reaction.

Other Transfusion Reactions

Infrequent immune transfusion reactions are listed in Table 5.1 and non-immunologic transfusion reactions are in Table 5.2.

References and Further Reading

Bruce JA, Kriese-Anderson L, Bruce AM, Pittman JR. (2015) Effect of premedication and other factors on the occurrence of acute transfusion reactions in dogs. *J Vet Emerg Crit Care* 25(5): 620–630.

Euler CC, Raj K, Mizukami K, Murray L, Chen CY, Mackin A, Giger U. (2016) Xenotransfusion of anemic cats with blood compatibility issues: pre- and posttransfusion laboratory diagnostic and crossmatching studies. *Vet Clin Pathol*. doi: 10.1111/vcp.12366 [Epub ahead of print]

Pennisi MG, Hartmann K, Addie DD, Lutz H, Gruffydd-Jones T, Boucraut-Baralon C, Egberink H, Frymus T, Horzinek MC, Hosie MJ, Lloret A, Marsilio F, Radford AD, Thiry E, Truyen U, Möstl K; European Advisory Board on Cat Diseases. (2015) Blood transfusion in cats: ABCD guidelines for minimizing risks of infectious iatrogenic complications. *J Feline Med Surg.* 17(7): 588–593.

Thomovsky EJ, Bach J. (2014) Incidence of acute lung injury in dogs receiving transfusions. *J Am Vet Med Assoc* 244(2): 170–174.

Weinstein NM. (2010) Transfusion reactions. In: *Schalm's Veterinary Hematology*, 6th edn. Weis DJ, Wardrop KJ, eds. Ames, IA: Wiley Blackwell.

Chapter 6 Methods and Storage

Introduction

Although there are often many different ways to perform the same task, standardization of procedures used for blood banking activities allows for reproducible test results and product safety and efficacy. The methods outlined in this chapter are examples of acceptable procedures; other adaptations of the same procedure may be used by facilities if desired. This chapter reviews blood typing methods and provides step-by-step procedures for compatibility testing and processing blood components.

Blood Typing

Blood type can be determined by several different methods. The "gold standard" of blood typing for dogs is detection of blood antigens by hemagglutination following incubation with polyclonal or monoclonal antibodies, while for cats the "gold standard" is the tube or microplate agglutination test. Since both of these methodologies are beyond the scope of clinical laboratories, this discussion is limited to "point-of-care" or "in-practice" assays that can be easily performed and provide quick and accurate results.

Canine

For routine component therapy, only DEA 1.1 blood type is determined. However, if the recipient is a potential transplant patient, is expected to have multiple transfusions, or has a non-regenerative erythrocyte disorder, full DEA testing should be performed for both the recipient and potential donors. Donors should be excluded if positive for 3, 5, and/or 7 (Hale, 2012).

Practical Transfusion Medicine for the Small Animal Practitioner, Second Edition. Carolyn A. Sink.
© 2017 John Wiley & Sons, Inc. Published 2017 by John Wiley & Sons, Inc.
Companion website: www.wiley.com/go/sink/transfusion

Card Method

DMS Laboratories offers an easy to use card-based method to determine DEA 1.1 status (RapidVet®-H Canine DEA 1.1 Blood Typing Agglutination Test Cards, dmslaboratories, inc., Flemington, NJ, USA). The assay is based on the agglutination reaction. A murine monoclonal antibody specific to DEA 1.1 is lyophilized on the test card and reconstituted with a diluent when ready for use. The newly formed antiserum reacts with patient erythrocytes when DEA 1.1 antigen is present on their surface. The results are visually identified by the presence of agglutination (Figure 6.1).

Membrane Diffusion Method

Alvedia offers an immunochromatographic test (QuickTEST DEA 1.1, Alvedia, Lyon, France). The test cartridge contains a membrane in which a monoclonal antibody to DEA 1.1 antigen has been embedded. Under the influence of a buffer flux, red blood cells migrate on the treated membrane via capillary action; retention of red cells (as a red cell band) at a designated point denotes the DEA 1 status of the test subject (Figure 6.2). Visualization of the control band verifies that the test ran successfully.

Automated Method

An automated method for blood typing is available outside the United States (QuickVet® Canine DEA 1.1™ Test, for use with the QuickVet® Analyzer, Scandinavian Micro Biodevices ApS, Denmark). The QuickVet® Diagnostic System consists of tabletop analyzer and single-use disposable test cartridges based on capillary-driven microfluidic technology (Figure 6.3).

Feline

In cats, determination of AB blood type is necessary for all cats at the time of transfusion because of the presence of naturally occurring alloantibodies.

Card Method

DMS Laboratories offers a card method to determine the blood type of cats (RapidVet®-H Feline Blood Typing Agglutination Test Cards, dmslaboratories, inc., Flemington, NJ, USA). The assay is based on the agglutination reaction of red cells. Lyophilized antisera in the two test wells of the card (the A-well contains murine monoclonal anti-A and the B-well contains *Triticum vulgaris* lectin) are reconstituted and mixed with patient whole blood; agglutination denotes a positive result (Figure 6.4).

Membrane Diffusion Method

Alvedia offers an immunochromatographic test (Quick Test A + B, Alvedia, Lyon, France). The test cartridge contains a membrane in which monoclonal antibodies specific to the A and B antigens are embedded. Under the influence of a buffer flux, red blood cells migrate on the treated membrane via capillary action; retention of red cells (as a red cell band) at a designated point determines if the

(a)

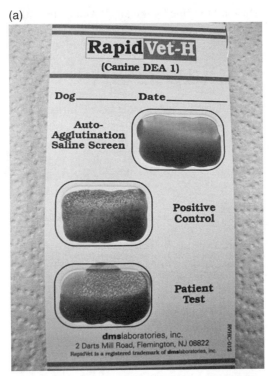

(b)

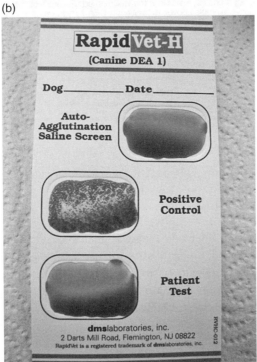

Figure 6.1 DMS RapidVet®-H Canine Blood Typing Test card: (a) DEA 1.1-positive, (b) DEA 1.1-negative, and (c) interpretation guide. Source: dmslaboratories, inc. Reproduced with permission.

(c)

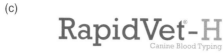

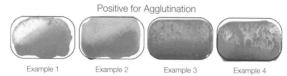

Canine Interpretation Guide

Positive for Agglutination

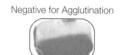

| Example 1 | Example 2 | Example 3 | Example 4 |

If the assay was run correctly, visible agglutination (see various positive examples above) should have occurred in the well marked Positive Control.

If the patient sample shows visible agglutination (see various positive examples above) in the well marked "Patient Test," the patient is DEA 1 positive. The "Auto-Agglutination Pre-Screen" well should not show agglutination. (Auto-agglutination is a rare occurrence.)

Negative for Agglutination

If no agglutination is visible in the well marked "Patient Test," (see negative example above), the patient is DEA 1 negative.

dmslaboratories, inc.
2 Darts Mill Road, Flemington, NJ 08822
Tel.: **(908) 782-3353** or **(800) 567-4367** in U.S. and Canada; Fax: **(908) 782-0832**
RapidVet is a registered trademark of **dms**laboratories, inc.

Figure 6.1 (Continued)

test subject is blood group A, B, or AB (Figure 6.5). Visualization of the control band verifies that the test ran successfully.

Automated Method

An automated method for blood typing is available outside the United States (QuickVet® Feline Blood Typing Test™, for use with the QuickVet® Analyzer, Scandinavian Micro Biodevices ApS, Denmark). The QuickVet® Diagnostic System consists of tabletop analyzer and single-use disposable test cartridges based on capillary-driven microfluidic technology.

Compatibility Testing

Crossmatches are performed to detect serologic incompatibilities. The methods described are limited to procedures that can easily be performed "in-practice" and will likely detect incompatibilities that could cause an acute or delayed hemolytic reaction.

The crossmatch is composed of three different tests:

- The major crossmatch is performed to detect antibodies in the recipient's plasma that may agglutinate or lyse the donor's erythrocytes.
- The minor crossmatch detects antibodies in the donor's plasma directed against the recipient's erythrocytes.
- The autocontrol can detect autoantibodies. It is run on both the patient and donor. A positive result warrants additional workup to investigate the cause.

Instructions for performing slide, tube, and gel-based crossmatch are found in Tables 6.1–6.3 and Figure 6.6. These procedures can be used for either dog or cat compatibility testing.

Selection of Blood Collection Systems

Collection systems are available in a variety of configurations, composed of a primary bag and satellite bags. The optimum blood draw volume is dependent on the blood collection system used. The draw volume is determined by the size of the bag and the amount of anticoagulant contained in the primary bag.

The needle is attached to the primary bag. The primary bag contains anticoagulant; the blood will flow directly into the primary bag during phlebotomy.

(a)

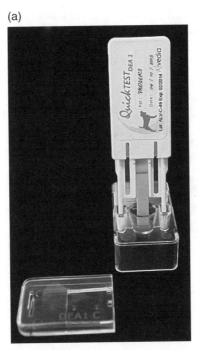

Figure 6.2 Alvedia QuickTEST. (a) DEA 1 (for dogs) and (b) interpretation guide. Source: Alvedia. Reproduced with permission.

(b)

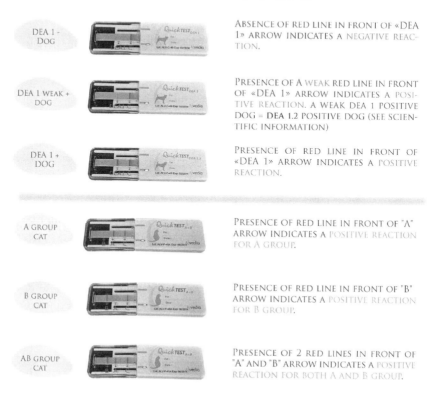

*Quick*TEST BT RESULTS

DEA 1 - DOG	ABSENCE OF RED LINE IN FRONT OF «DEA 1» ARROW INDICATES A NEGATIVE REACTION.
DEA 1 WEAK + DOG	PRESENCE OF A WEAK RED LINE IN FRONT OF «DEA 1» ARROW INDICATES A POSITIVE REACTION. A WEAK DEA 1 POSITIVE DOG = **DEA 1.2 POSITIVE DOG** (SEE SCIENTIFIC INFORMATION)
DEA 1 + DOG	PRESENCE OF RED LINE IN FRONT OF «DEA 1» ARROW INDICATES A POSITIVE REACTION.
A GROUP CAT	PRESENCE OF RED LINE IN FRONT OF "A" ARROW INDICATES A POSITIVE REACTION FOR A GROUP.
B GROUP CAT	PRESENCE OF RED LINE IN FRONT OF "B" ARROW INDICATES A POSITIVE REACTION FOR B GROUP.
AB GROUP CAT	PRESENCE OF 2 RED LINES IN FRONT OF "A" AND "B" ARROW INDICATES A POSITIVE REACTION FOR BOTH A AND B GROUP.

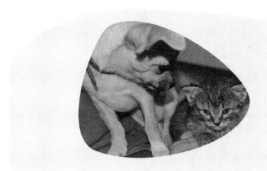

Figure 6.2 (Continued)

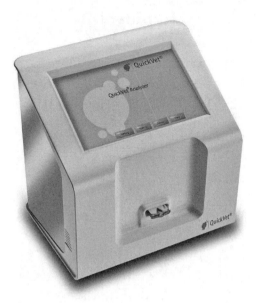

Figure 6.3 QuickVet® Diagnostic System. Source: Scandinavian Micro Biodevices ApS, Denmark. Reproduced with permission.

(a)

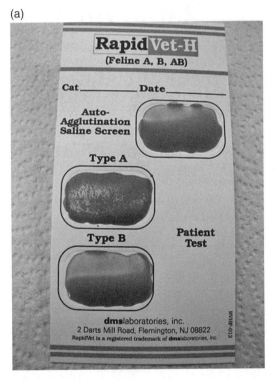

Figure 6.4 DMS RapidVet®-H Feline Blood Typing Test card. (a) Type A, (b) type B, and (c) interpretation guide. Source: dmslaboratories, inc. Reproduced with permission.

(b)

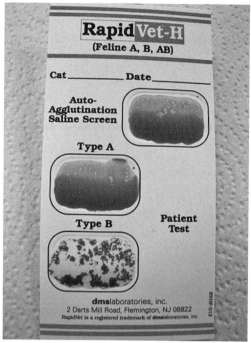

(c)

RapidVet®-H
Feline Blood Typing

Feline Interpretation Guide

Positive for Agglutination

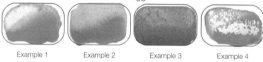

| Example 1 | Example 2 | Example 3 | Example 4 |

If the assay was run correctly, visible agglutination (see various positive examples above) should have occurred in at least one of the wells marked "Patient Test." The "Auto-Agglutination Pre-Screen" well should not show agglutination. (Auto-agglutination is a rare occurrence.)

If the patient sample shows agglutination in the well marked "Type A," the cat tested has blood group A. In this case, the well marked "Type B" will be negative for agglutination. (See negative example below.)

If the patient sample shows agglutination in the well marked "Type B," the cat tested has blood group B. In this case, the well marked "Type A" will be negative for agglutination.

If the patient sample shows agglutination in both patient wells, the cat tested has blood group AB.

Negative for Agglutination

dmslaboratories, inc.
2 Darts Mill Road, Flemington, NJ 08822
Tel.: **(908) 782-3353** or **(800) 567-4367** in U.S. and Canada; Fax: **(908) 782-0832**
RapidVet is a registered trademark of **dms**laboratories, inc.

Figure 6.4 (Continued)

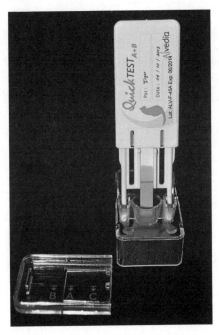

Figure 6.5 Alvedia QuickTEST A+B (for cats). Source: Alvedia. Reproduced with permission.

Table 6.1 Procedure for tube crossmatch

Specimens
- Anticoagulated (EDTA, heparin, or citrate) whole blood from the recipient; EDTA-anticoagulated blood is preferred. (Note: Serum may be used instead of plasma, but should NOT be obtained from serum separator.)
- One of the following:
  - o Individual segments from banked donor blood bags
  - o Anticoagulated (EDTA, heparin, or citrate) whole blood from a potential donor; EDTA-anticoagulated blood is preferred.

Materials and equipment
- 37 °C incubator
- Normal saline
- 12 × 75 mm glass test tubes
- Disposable pipettes
- Baxter Immufuge II Centrifuge (tube centrifuge) (Note: The Baxter Immufuge II is automatically pre-set to run within a range of 3075–3375 rpm with no brake at room temperature.)
- Microscope
- Scissors

Procedure
A. Selection of donor blood for crossmatching
1. Dogs and cats should be blood typed prior to crossmatching.
2. For banked blood: Ensure that any banked blood product is within the expiration date on the product label. Do not use a blood product that is expired.
3. Obtain type-specific donor units or a blood specimen from a type-specific potential donor matching the recipient for the crossmatch procedure:

(Continued)

Table 6.1 (Continued)

Recipient blood type	Column A Preferred donor unit	Column B Preferred donor unit if column A unit is not available	Column C Preferred donor unit if column A or B unit is not available
DEA 1.1 (−)	DEA 1.1 (−)	Universal	Consult clinician
DEA 1.1 (+)	DEA 1.1 (+)	DEA 1.1 (−)	Universal
Feline type A	Feline type A	Consult clinician	
Feline type B	Feline type B	Consult clinician	
Feline type AB	Feline type A	Feline type B or AB	Consult clinician

B. Separate the red blood cells and plasma

1. For banked donor blood:
   a. Obtain one segment from each donor blood bag and place them into a labeled 12 × 75 mm glass test tube.
   b. Centrifuge the segments for 1 minute in the tube centrifuge to separate the plasma from the red cells.
   c. Carefully cut the segment at the plasma/red cell junction with scissors. (Clean the scissors after each cut to avoid cross-contamination of segments.)
   d. Gently squeeze the red cells and plasma into separately labeled 12 × 75 mm glass test tubes.
2. For recipient blood and non-banked donor blood:
   a. Aliquot a small amount of patient EDTA whole blood into a labeled 12 × 75 mm glass test tube.
   b. Centrifuge the sample for 3 minutes in the tube centrifuge.
   c. Using a disposable pipette, remove the plasma from the red cells and place the plasma into a separate, properly labeled 12 × 75 mm glass test tube. Save the red cells for the next step.

C. Prepare the donor and patient red cell suspensions

1. Add normal saline to the donor and recipient red cells in the tube and gently mix by pipetting the mixture up and down a few times.
2. Centrifuge for 1 minute in the tube centrifuge.
3. Decant and discard the supernatant into a biohazard waste container.
4. Repeat steps C1 through C3 at least two more times, for a total of three or more washes.
5. After the last wash, decant and discard the supernatant into a biohazard waste container. Centrifuge the red cells for 15 seconds in the tube centrifuge to make a packed cell button. Prepare a 3% red blood cell (RBC) suspension for the patient and each donor by adding 50 μl of packed red blood cells from the red cell button to 2000 μl of normal saline.

D. Crossmatch procedure

1. Label the tubes with the appropriate information, which includes patient ID, donor ID, autocontrol, major, and/or minor.
2. Add the plasma/serum and red cell suspensions (from section B) to the labeled wells as described below:

Test	Cell suspension (1 drop)	Plasma/serum (2 drops)
Patient autocontrol	Patient	Patient
Major crossmatch	Donor	Patient
Minor crossmatch	Patient	Donor
Donor autocontrol	Donor	Donor

Table 6.1 (Continued)

3. Mix all the tubes (by gently shaking) and incubate in the 37 °C incubator for 15 minutes.
4. Centrifuge for 15 seconds in the tube centrifuge.
5. Gently remove samples from centrifuge without disturbing the cell buttons.
6. Grade the reactions.
7. Evaluate the samples for hemolysis by evaluating the supernatants for red discoloration:

Crossmatch	Compare supernatant to:	Result and interpretation
Major	Patient plasma (or patient AC supernatant)	a. Patient's plasma and supernatant similar red intensity and red blood cell particulates are present: • Origin of hemolysis is patient's plasma • Crossmatch is negative for hemolysis b. Supernatant is more red than patient's plasma and red blood cell particulates are absent: • Origin of hemolysis is the crossmatch • Crossmatch is positive for hemolysis
Minor	Donor plasma (or donor AC supernatant)	a. Donor's plasma and supernatant similar red intensity and red blood cell particulates are present: • Origin of hemolysis is donor's plasma • Crossmatch is negative for hemolysis b. Supernatant is more red than donor's plasma and red blood cell particulates are absent: • Origin of hemolysis is the crossmatch • Crossmatch is positive for hemolysis

8. Evaluate the samples for agglutination:
    a. Holding the tube in a well-lit area, preferably with a white background, gently shake the tube to disrupt the red cell button. This movement should gently move the supernatant back and forth over the cell button using a shaking or tilting motion.
    b. Observe the manner in which the red blood cells leave the red cell button.
9. Read macroscopically and microscopically. Grade the reaction using the following guidelines:

Macro 4+	One solid aggregate of cells
Macro 3+	Several large aggregates
Macro 2+	Large agglutinates and smaller clumps
Macro 1+	Many small agglutinates and a background free of red cells
Micro	No agglutinates seen macroscopically; agglutinates seen microscopically
No reaction	Negative. No agglutination observed macroscopically or microscopically

(Continued)

Table 6.1 (Continued)

Reaction grading

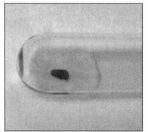

4+ Reaction

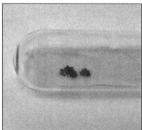

3+ Reaction

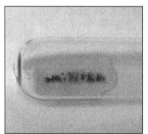

2+ Reaction

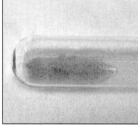

1+ Reaction

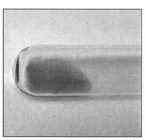

Negative reaction

10. The presence or absence of rouleaux may be confirmed using the following saline replacement procedure: Red blood cells exhibiting rouleaux appear as "stacked coins" when observed microscopically. Rouleaux formations disperse with the addition of normal saline while true agglutination remains. For compatibility testing, rouleaux is considered a negative reaction. The following procedure is used to distinguish rouleaux from true agglutination. If rouleaux is suspected:

   a. Re-centrifuge the sample for 15 seconds and decant the serum/plasma from the 12 × 75 mm tube.
   b. To the cell button, add 2 drops of saline. Mix by gentle shaking until the cell button is re-suspended.
   c. Centrifuge the sample for 15 seconds.
   d. Grade the reaction as outlined in step D9 above.

E. Results and reporting
- True rouleaux will disperse with the addition of saline and is not considered agglutination.
- Autocontrol, major crossmatch, minor crossmatch are reported as:
   o Compatible: No reaction or
   o Incompatible: Hemolysis, 4+, 3+, 2+, 1+, or Micro.

F. Test limitations
- False positive or false negative test results can occur from bacterial or chemical contamination of testing materials, inadequate incubation time or temperature, improper centrifugation, improper storage of materials, or omission of test samples.

Source: Virginia Tech Animal Laboratory Services (2015).

Table 6.2 Slide crossmatch

Specimens

- Anticoagulated (EDTA, heparin, or citrate) whole blood from the recipient; EDTA-anticoagulated blood is preferred. (Note: Serum may be used instead of plasma, but should NOT be obtained from serum separator.)
- One of the following:
  o Individual segments from banked donor blood bags
  o Anticoagulated (EDTA, heparin, or citrate) whole blood from a potential donor; EDTA-anticoagulated blood is preferred.

Procedure

1. Centrifuge and separate specimens into cells and plasma or serum.
2. Label four glass slides as Major, Minor, Donor AC, and Patient AC.
3. Dispense specimens as listed below:

Test	Red blood cells (1 drop)	Plasma or serum (2 drops)
Major crossmatch	Donor	Patient
Minor crossmatch	Patient	Donor
Donor autocontrol	Donor	Donor
Patient autocontrol	Patient	Patient

4. Mix samples with an applicator stick. Be sure to use a fresh stick on each slide to avoid cross-contamination.
5. Gently rock the slides.
6. After 2 minutes, observe the slides for macroscopic agglutination.
7. Place a coverslip on the slide and view the red cells microscopically using a 40× objective.

Results and reporting

- Any agglutination is considered a positive reaction.

Other smaller bags, which are integrally attached to the primary bag through sealed ports, are the satellite bags. There may be one or more satellite bags depending on the configuration of the blood collection system used (Figure 6.7).

For dogs, 450 ml blood collection systems can be used. For cats, a specialized blood collection system can be used (Figure 6.8).

Pre-processing Guidelines

All blood products should be labeled with the phlebotomy date, product name, and expiration date. Additional information such as the blood type and donor identification is necessary. Permanent markers should be used for labeling so that this information is not washed off during storage, thawing, or warming of the product.

Before processing begins, the needle should be removed from the blood collection system. This is accomplished by heat-seal or metal clips.

Table 6.3 Procedure for gel crossmatch using DiaMed Products

Specimens

- Anticoagulated (EDTA, heparin, or citrate) whole blood from the recipient; EDTA-anticoagulated blood is preferred. (Note: Serum may be used instead of plasma, but should NOT be obtained from serum separator.)
- One of the following:
  - o Individual segments from banked donor blood bags
  - o Anticoagulated (EDTA, heparin, or citrate) whole blood from a potential donor; EDTA-anticoagulated blood is preferred.

Materials and equipment

- Micro typing gel card
- MTS Diluent 2
- MTS 0.5 ml Dispenser™
- 10 µl, 25 µl, 50 µl pipettes
- Pipette tips
- Normal saline (fresh)
- 12 × 75 mm glass test tubes
- Disposable pipettes
- DiaMed-ID Incubator 37 SI (37 °C gel card incubator)
- DiaMed-ID Centrifuge 6S (gel card centrifuge) (Note: The DiaMed-ID Centrifuge 6S is automatically pre-set to run within a range of 1165–1185 rpm with no brake at room temperature.)
- Baxter Immufuge II Centrifuge (tube centrifuge) (Note: The Baxter Immufuge II is automatically pre-set to run within a range of 3075–3375 rpm with no brake at room temperature.)
- Scissors

Procedure
A. Selection of donor blood for crossmatch

1. Dogs and cats should be blood typed prior to crossmatch.
2. Obtain type-specific donor units matching the recipient for the crossmatch procedure. Use the following table to choose the correct unit(s) for the recipient:

Recipient blood type	Column A Preferred donor unit	Column B Preferred donor unit if column A unit is not available	Column C Preferred donor unit if column A or B unit is not available
DEA 1.1 (−)	DEA 1.1 (−)	Universal	Consult clinician
DEA 1.1 (+)	DEA 1.1 (+)	DEA 1.1 (−)	Universal
Feline type A	Feline type A	Consult clinician	
Feline type B	Feline type B	Consult clinician	
Feline type AB	Feline type A	Feline type B or AB	Consult clinician

3. Ensure that any banked blood product is within the expiration date on the product label. Do not use a blood product that is expired.
4. For non-banked blood (direct from a potential donor), utilize the blood sample(s) collected directly from the potential donor.

B. Prepare reagents

1. Remove the MTS Diluent 2 from the refrigerator and allow it to warm to room temperature.
2. Ensure that the normal saline is fresh by obtaining a clean squeeze bottle and pouring fresh normal saline into the bottle before beginning the procedure.

Table 6.3 (Continued)

C. Prepare donor and patient samples

1. Prepare the patient 0.8% red cell suspension and plasma:
   a. Aliquot a small amount of patient EDTA whole blood into a labeled 12 × 75 mm glass test tube.
   b. Centrifuge the sample for 3 minutes in the tube centrifuge.
   c. Using a disposable pipette, remove the plasma from the cell button and place the plasma into a separate, properly labeled 12 × 75 mm glass test tube.
   d. Wash the remaining red cells with normal saline: Add normal saline to the red cells in tube and mix gently by pipetting the mixture up and down a few times.
   e. Centrifuge for 1 minute in the tube centrifuge.
   f. Decant and discard the supernatant into a red biohazard waste container.
   g. Repeat steps d–f two more times, for a total of three or more washes.
   h. After the last wash, decant and discard the supernatant into a biohazard waste container.
   i. Centrifuge the red cells for 15 seconds in the tube centrifuge to make a packed cell button.
   j. Using the MTS 0.5 ml Dispenser™, dispense 1 ml (2 pumps) of MTS Diluent 2 into a clean 12 × 75 mm glass test tube labeled with the recipient information.
   k. Add 10 μl of recipient packed red cells from the red cell button to the labeled tube with the MTS Diluent and mix gently by pipetting the mixture up and down a few times.
2. Prepare the donor 0.8% red cell suspension and plasma. For banked donor blood use all steps a–l; for non-banked donor blood follow steps d–l but use the donor's EDTA whole blood.
   a. Remove the individual segment from donor blood bag and place into a labeled 12 × 75 mm glass test tube.
   b. Centrifuge the segment for 1 minute in the tube centrifuge to separate the plasma from the red cells.
   c. Carefully cut the segment at the plasma/red cell junction with scissors. (Clean the scissors after each cut to avoid cross-contamination of segments.)
   d. Gently squeeze the red cells and plasma into separately labeled 12 × 75 mm glass test tubes.
   e. Wash the red cells with normal saline: Add normal saline to the red cells in tube and mix gently by pipetting the mixture up and down a few times.
   f. Centrifuge for 1 minute in the tube centrifuge.
   g. Decant and discard the supernatant into a biohazard waste container.
   h. Repeat steps e–g two or more times, for a total of three or more washes.
   i. After the last wash, decant and discard the supernatant into a biohazard waste container.
   j. Centrifuge the red cells for 15 seconds in the tube centrifuge to make a packed cell button.
   k. Dispense 1 ml (2 pumps) of MTS Diluent 2 into a clean 12 × 75 mm glass test tube labeled with the donor information.
   l. Add 10 μl of donor packed red cells from the red cell button to the labeled tube with MTS Diluent and mix gently by pipetting the mixture up and down a few times.

D. Crossmatch procedure

1. Inspect the gel columns on the gel card for bubbles or drying. Bubbles may be remedied by centrifugation in the gel card centrifuge but dried gel columns should not be used.
2. Appropriately label sections on the gel card with the appropriate information, which may include patient ID, donor ID, autocontrol (AC), major (M), and/or minor (m).
3. Remove the foil from the gel card by holding the gel card in an upward position. Only remove enough foil for the number of columns needed for testing.
4. Add the 0.8% red cell suspensions and serum/plasma to labeled wells as described below:

Test	Cell suspension (1 drop)	Plasma/serum (2 drops)
Patient autocontrol	Patient	Patient
Major crossmatch	Donor	Patient
Minor crossmatch	Patient	Donor
Donor autocontrol	Donor	Donor

(Continued)

Table 6.3 (Continued)

5. Incubate the gel card in the DiaMed-ID Incubator 37 SI for 15 minutes at 37 °C.
6. Centrifuge the gel card for 10 minutes in the gel card centrifuge.
7. Grade the reactions.
8. Evaluate the samples for hemolysis by evaluating the supernatants for red discoloration:

Crossmatch	Compare supernatant to:	Result and interpretation
Major	Patient plasma (or patient AC supernatant)	a. Patient's plasma and supernatant similar red intensity and red blood cell particulates are present: • Origin of hemolysis is patient's plasma • Crossmatch is negative for hemolysis b. Supernatant is more red than patient's plasma and red blood cell particulates are absent: • Origin of hemolysis is the crossmatch • Crossmatch is positive for hemolysis.
Minor	Donor plasma (or donor AC supernatant)	a. Donor's plasma and supernatant similar red intensity and red blood cell particulates are present: • Origin of hemolysis is donor's plasma • Crossmatch is negative for hemolysis b. Supernatant is more red than donor's plasma and red blood cell particulates are absent: • Origin of hemolysis is the crossmatch • Crossmatch is positive for hemolysis

9. Evaluate the samples for agglutination:

Grade	Description
4+ Agglutination	Solid band of red blood cell agglutinates on top of the gel. A few agglutinates may filter into the gel but remain near the predominant band
3+ Agglutination	The majority of red blood cell agglutinates are trapped in the upper half of the gel microtube
2+ Agglutination	Red blood cell agglutinates are dispersed throughout the length of the gel microtube. Few unagglutinated red blood cells may be observed in the bottom of the microtube
1+ Agglutination	Red blood cell agglutinates are observed predominantly in the lower half of the gel microtube. Unagglutinated red blood cells form a button in the bottom of the microtube
0 Negative	Unagglutinated red blood cells form a well-defined button at the bottom of the microtube
Mixed Field (MF)	Red blood cell agglutinates at the top of the gel or dispersed throughout the gel microtube accompanied by a button of negative red blood cells in the bottom of the microtube. NOTE: This reaction should be further evaluated to be either a true positive (3+) reaction or a false positive result due to clots, particulates, or other artifacts within the sample

Table 6.3 (Continued)

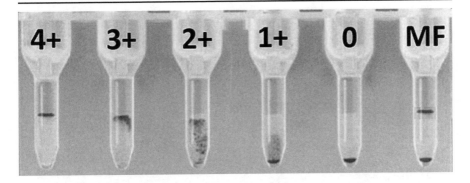

10. If a positive reaction is observed on the minor crossmatch, perform a donor autocontrol, and record the results on the unit.

E. Results and reporting

- Autocontrol, major crossmatch, minor crossmatch are reported as:
  - o Compatible: negative or
  - o Incompatible: Hemolysis, 4+, 3+, 2+ or 1+.

F. Test limitations

- False positive or false negative test results can occur from bacterial or chemical contamination of testing materials, inadequate incubation time or temperature, improper centrifugation, improper storage of materials, or omission of test samples.
- False positive results may occur if a card that shows signs of drying is used in testing.
- Red blood cells must be diluted with the appropriate diluent at the proper concentration before addition to the gel card. Variations in cell concentration can markedly affect the sensitivity of test results.
- Hemolyzed and grossly icteric blood samples may be difficult to visually interpret in the gel and therefore test results should not be used.
- Anomalous results may be caused by fibrin or other particulate matter in blood samples that could stick to the sides of the microtube.
- Aged or hemolyzed blood may yield weaker reactions than those obtained with fresh red blood cells.
- Antibodies to preservatives, medications, disease states, and/or cross-contamination of reaction microtubes may cause false positive reactions.

Source: Virginia Tech Animal Laboratory Services (2015).

Once the needle is removed, the phlebotomy line should be cleared using a tube stripper; this will assure that the line is properly anticoagulated. This is important because this line will now be separated into segments that will be used as the donor blood sample for compatibility testing (Figure 6.9).

Each 450 ml blood bag has a set of identification numbers repeated the length of the blood collection line. Place the first seal after the first identification number that is located at the top of the blood bag and repeat sealing segments for the length of the phlebotomy line. If no identifiers are on the blood collection line, heat-seal segments approximately 3–4 cm long. Fold the segments end to end and rubber band them together: this will prevent the segments from getting tangled in the centrifuge head if the unit is processed for components.

(a)

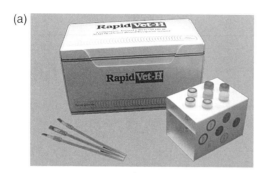

(b)

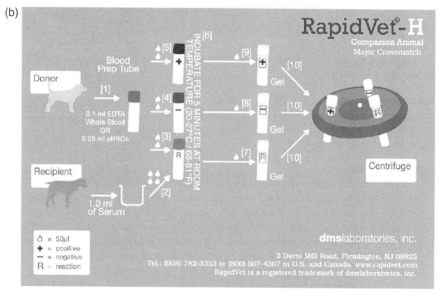

(c)

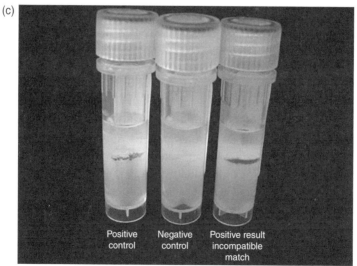

Figure 6.6 DMS RapidVet®-H. (a) Companion Animal Major Crossmatch Kit, (b) instructions, and (c) interpretation. Source: dmslaboratories, inc. Reproduced with permission.

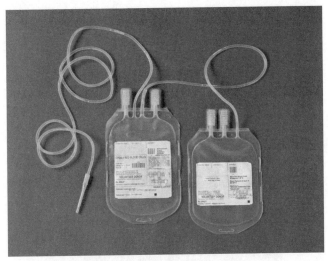

Figure 6.7 A 450 ml blood collection system with satellite bags. Source: Animal Blood Resources International. Used with permission.

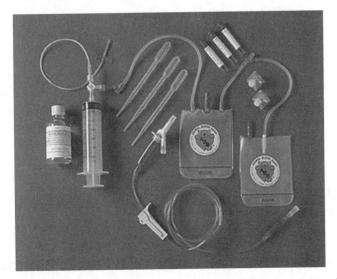

Figure 6.8 Blood collection bag for cats. Source: Animal Blood Resources International. Reproduced with permission.

If segments are inadvertently separated from the blood bag during storage, the identification number on the segments can be compared to the identification number on the blood bag.

Preparation of Fresh Whole Blood

Canine

Once a unit of whole blood has been collected, it should be stored at 1–6 °C until processing is possible unless it will be used to produce platelet preparations.

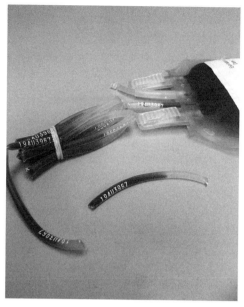

Figure 6.9 Heat-sealed segments for use in compatibility testing.

A unit of whole blood is considered fresh whole blood for a time period of 24 hours after the phlebotomy. Fresh whole blood contains all blood elements.

If absolutely no components will be processed from the unit of fresh whole blood, the satellite bags may be sealed from the primary bag, detached, and discarded.

Feline

When a syringe or bag of feline whole blood is collected in an open system, it should be transfused as soon as possible. If significant delays are imminent, store the product at 1–6 °C until transfusion is possible.

Preparation of Red Cells and Fresh Frozen Plasma

Canine

This discussion is limited to 450 ml blood collection for dogs.

When the blood collection process is complete, a unit of whole blood should be stored at 1–6 °C until component preparation is possible.

If the component fresh frozen plasma is to be made, the plasma must be separated from the red cells and completely frozen within 8 hours of collection if the anticoagulant–preservative is CPD, CP2D, or CPDA-1. If the anticoagulant is ACD, separation and freezing must occur within 6 hours of phlebotomy.

Whole blood designated for platelet preparations should remain at room temperature until the platelets are removed.

Preparation for Centrifugation

The entire unit of blood should be weighed. This weight is used exclusively for balancing the centrifuge.

Proper centrifuge balance is important to prevent wear of the centrifuge rotor; total weight in opposing cups should be equal.

An empty blood bag may be filled with 10% glycerin in order to provide an equally weighted balance bag for centrifugation, Rubber bands and weighted plastic discs can be added to the bottom of the centrifuge cup to achieve balance.

Centrifugation

Blood bags should be placed in the centrifuge bucket with the label facing out. This reduces the centrifugal force on sealed margins of the blood bag. Centrifuges with swinging cups provide for easier separation of the plasma from the red cells (because the meniscus is horizontal).

The unit of whole blood should be centrifuged using a heavy spin in a refrigerated centrifuge between 1 and 6 °C. A heavy spin is defined as $5000g$ for 5 minutes. For calibration of the centrifuge, the calculation for relative centrifugal force (RCF) is given by:

$$RCF(in\ g) = 28.38 \times radius\ of\ centrifuge\ rotor\ in\ inches \times (rpm\ /\ 1000)^2$$

where rpm is revolutions per minute, which can be verified by a tachometer.

Once centrifugation has ceased, it is important to allow the centrifuge to stop spinning without assistance, as brake use or an acute stop of the rotor will disturb the red cell/plasma separation, thus contaminating the plasma with red cells.

Component Separation

The unit of blood should be removed from the centrifuge without agitation so as not to disturb the red cells and plasma. The unit is then placed on a plasma extractor. This piece of equipment provides a rigid stand in which to place a unit of whole blood; a hinged plate is attached to the stand and may be released to apply pressure to the unit of whole blood in order to express the plasma into a satellite bag. For this discussion, there are two satellite bags: one contains a red cell additive and the other is empty. Note that the number of satellite bags depends on the blood collection system being used.

Place the empty satellite bag on a balance that has been tared to zero. Express the plasma into the empty bag. Remove 230–256 g of plasma.

Using hemostats, clamp off the line of the bag containing the harvested plasma. Then, break the seal from the additive bag and let the additive flow into the red cells. Seal the bag containing the red cells and additive and remove the red cell bag from the plasma bags. Gently mix the red cells and additive.

Two satellite bags remain; one contains 230–256 g of plasma with a volume of 225–250 ml. The plasma may be left in one bag or divided into volumes as needed. Seal the plasma bag(s) as appropriate.

The choice to divide the plasma should be made based on typical recipient size and plasma demand. Blood collection systems may be purchased with one to four satellite bags and should be selected for use accordingly.

Tare the weight of the balance to zero and weigh each of the filled blood bags. Subtract the weight of the empty bag from the final weight of the filled bag. The specific gravity of red cells is 1.080–1.090; the specific gravity of plasma is 1.023. By dividing the final weight of the product by the appropriate specific gravity, the volume of the product in milliliters can be calculated.

The final product should be labeled with the product name and volume in milliliters. If additive has been added to the red cells, this should be noted on the bag.

Feline
Preparation
The unit of whole blood is stored at 2–6 °C until component preparation is possible. The plasma must be separated from the red cells and completely frozen within 8 hours of collection when the anticoagulant is CPDA.

Re-strip the blood collection line with the tubing stripper and heat-seal the stripped blood collection line into segments. Each blood bag has identifying numbers on the blood collection line. Place the first seal after the first identification number that is located at the top of the blood bag, beside the ports. Then clip the line after the last segment, detaching the syringe that is used to draw the unit.

Fold the segments end to end and rubber band them together.

Centrifugation
Place the unit and satellite bags into a centrifuge bucket; pack the unit securely into the bucket using foam pads or other material.

Use the balance to determine the weight of the bucket and unit. This weight is used exclusively for balancing the centrifuge.

If there are an odd number of units to be centrifuged, balance the centrifuge by using blood bags filled with 10% glycerin. Rubber bands and weighted plastic discs can be used to even out smaller weight discrepancies. If there is an even number of units to be centrifuged, balance the units using the weighted plastic discs to even out the weight discrepancies between buckets.

Centrifuge the blood bag(s) with the label facing out. This reduces the centrifugal force on sealed margins.

Centrifuge for 3 minutes at 2 °C at 2000 rpm. DO NOT use the brake to stop the centrifuge.

Plasma Extraction
Remove the unit of blood from the centrifuge so as not to disturb red cells and plasma. Place the empty satellite bag on the balance and tare to zero.

Break the seal in the top of the satellite bag. Use the plasma extractor or manual pressure with blocks on each side of the bag to express 20 g of plasma into the satellite bag (1 ml = 1 g plasma). Since the volume of plasma is small and the extraction goes quickly, this step may require the assistance of another technician.

Using hemostats, clamp the line between the packed red cell unit and the plasma unit. Heat-seal or use metal clamps to separate the red blood cell bag and the plasma bag. Discard any excessive tubing.

Weighing

Tare the weight of the balance to zero and weigh each of the filled blood bags. Subtract the weight of the empty bag from the final weight of the filled bag. The specific gravity of red cells is 1.080–1.090; the specific gravity of plasma is 1.023. By dividing the final weight of the product by the appropriate specific gravity, the volume of the product in milliliters can be calculated.

The final product should be labeled with the product name and species.

Labeling

Label the packed cell unit with the collection date, unit number, expiration date, volume (in milliliters), blood type, and any additive used. Labeling may be done by hand-writing, using permanent marker, or by using an appropriate pre-printed label.

Label the plasma unit with the collection date, donor identification, expiration date (1 year from the date of phlebotomy), species, volume (in milliliters), blood type, and any additive used. Labeling may be done by hand-writing, using permanent marker, or by using an appropriate pre-printed label.

Storage

Store packed feline red cells at 2–6 °C. The feline stock should be segregated from the canine stock.

Feline plasma products should be stored at –18 °C or below and segregated from the canine stock.

Cryoprecipitate and Cryo-Poor Plasma, Canine only

Cryoprecipitated anti-hemophilic factor and cryo-poor plasma are made from 1 unit of FFP. To process cryoprecipitated anti-hemophilic factor from FFP, a full unit (225–250 ml) of FFP with at least one integrally attached satellite bag is needed. FFP should be processed as outlined in the procedure above except the entire unit of FFP should remain in one satellite bag.

It is important to document the total volume of the unit of FFP as this value will be used in a subsequent calculation.

The line between two satellite bags should be temporarily occluded in order to prevent transfer of plasma to the second satellite bag. The FFP should be frozen solid before preparing the cryoprecipitated anti-hemophilic factor.

Allow the unit of FFP to thaw at 1–6 °C, which takes about 8 hours. When the plasma has a slushy consistency, harvest the cryoprecipitated anti-hemophilic factor using one of the two following methods.

- Place the thawing plasma in a plasma extractor. Express the liquid plasma into the empty integrally attached satellite bag. The newly filled satellite bag should contain 90% of the original volume of FFP. Seal both bags.

OR

- Centrifuge the bag using a heavy spin. The cryoprecipitated anti-hemophilic factor will precipitate and adhere to the sides of the bag. Express 90% of the supernatant into the empty satellite bag. Seal both bags.

The newly filled satellite bag containing 90% of the FFP is now cryo-poor plasma. The satellite bag containing the residual 10% of the FFP is cryoprecipitated anti-hemophilic factor.

Freeze the cryoprecipitated anti-hemophilic factor and cryo-poor plasma within 1 hour of completion of preparation. Both products should be stored at −18 °C or lower. Product expiration is one year from the date of phlebotomy (not the date of preparation).

The product should be labeled with product name, species, total volume, and expiration date.

Preparation of Platelet Concentrates, Canine Only

Preparation of Platelet-Rich Plasma
Platelet-rich plasma (PRP) is made from one unit of fresh whole blood (450 ml draw). To prepare PRP, a unit of fresh whole blood with at least one integrally attached satellite bag is needed. The unit of fresh whole blood should be maintained at 22–25 °C and processed immediately in order to harvest viable platelets.

Preparation for Centrifugation
The entire unit of blood should be weighed. This weight is used exclusively for balancing the centrifuge. Proper centrifuge balance is important to prevent wear of the centrifuge rotor; total weight in opposing cups should be equal. An empty blood bag may be filled with 10% glycerin in order to provide an equally weighted balance bag for centrifugation. Rubber bands and weighted plastic discs can be added to the bottom of the centrifuge cup to achieve balance.

The unit of whole blood should be centrifuged using a light spin in a centrifuge at 22–25 °C. (A light spin is defined as 200 g for 3 minutes.)

Once centrifugation has ceased, it is important to allow the centrifuge to stop spinning without assistance, as brake use or an acute stop of the rotor will disturb the red cell/plasma separation, thus contaminating the plasma with red cells.

Component Separation

The unit of blood should be removed from the centrifuge without agitation so as not to disturb the red cells and plasma. The unit is placed on a plasma extractor, which provides a rigid stand in which to place a unit of whole blood. A hinged plate is attached to the stand and may be released to apply pressure to the unit of whole blood in order to express the plasma into a satellite bag.

Place the empty satellite bag on a balance that has been tared to zero. Remove plasma.

The task of extracting platelets from centrifuged whole blood can be challenging as red cells lie just below the platelet layer. PRP should be light yellow in color and should not contain visible red cell contamination.

Using hemostats, clamp off the line of the bag containing the harvested plasma and seal. Process the red cells as described earlier.

To calculate the volume of PRP, first tare the weight of the balance to zero and weigh the PRP. Substract the weight of the empty bag from the final weight of the bag. The specific gravity of plasma is 1.023, so 1 g of plasma is approximately equal to 1 ml of plasma. By dividing the final weight of the product by the appropriate specific gravity, the volume of product in milliliters can be calculated. The final product should be labeled with the product name and volume in milliliters.

Storage

In order to preserve platelet viability, PRP should be allowed to "rest" at room temperature, label side down, for 1–2 hours and transfused as soon as possible thereafter.

Short Draw and Decreasing the Amount of Anticoagulant–Preservative, Canine Only

Commercially available blood bags are designed to anticoagulate and preserve a specific amount of blood. Deviations from the expected blood volume must be handled appropriately in order to assure product viability. This discussion will be limited to those bags designed for a 450 ml draw, although the principles may be applied to bags with different expected draw volumes.

Short Draw

Blood collection bags intended for a 450 ml draw contain approximately 63 ml of anticoagulant–preservative. This amount of anticoagulant–preservative is sufficient to support 405–495 ml of whole blood. If 300–404 ml of whole blood is drawn into a bag intended for a 450 ml draw, the unit of blood should not be processed into components and should remain as whole blood. The unit of blood should be labeled as "Short Draw" and the volume of the draw should be documented on the bag.

Decreasing the Amount of Anticoagulant–Preservative

If a phlebotomy of less than 300 ml is planned, the amount of anticoagulant–preservative in the blood bag should be decreased prior to collection. Anticoagulant–preservative may be removed by expressing the excess anticoagulant–preservative solution into one of the integrally attached satellite bags (see Table 3.1).

Procedure for Removal of Anticoagulant–Preservative from the Primary Blood Bag

Obtain the specific gravity and amount of the anticoagulant–preservative in the primary bag. Calculate the weight of the anticoagulant–preservative to be removed from the primary bag.

Weigh both the primary bag and the satellite bag designated for collection of excess anticoagulant–preservative.

Open the port from the primary bag. Express the calculated amount of anticoagulant–preservative to be removed into the empty satellite bag. Seal and remove the satellite bag.

The unit may be processed for components.

Storage of Blood Products

Red cells should be refrigerated at 1–6 °C. While a refrigerator dedicated to blood storage is ideal, there are a variety of refrigerators available in a wide price range that will maintain adequate temperature. The blood product should be stored in an organized fashion. It is advantageous to place the shortest date (the unit that expires first) at the front of the refrigerator so that it will be used first. Other products or supplies that may be stored in the same refrigerator should be segregated from the units of red cells.

Plasma products other than platelets should be stored at −18 °C or below. A freezer dedicated to plasma storage is optimal. Freezers used to store plasma products should not possess defrost cycles that compromise product storage temperature.

To monitor stored plasma for inadvertent thawing, one of two techniques may be utilized.

• Place a rubber band around the middle of a unit of plasma before it is frozen. When the product is frozen, remove the rubber band, leaving a "waist" indentation on the unit. If the unit thaws, the waist disappears. Thus, a unit of plasma removed from the freezer without the waist indentation has likely been warmed above freezing during storage.

OR

• Turn the unit upsidedown before freezing. This creates a "bubble" on the bottom of the plasma bag. Once frozen, the bag should be placed upright. If the unit of plasma is removed from the freezer and does not have a bubble in the bottom of the bag, it has likely been warmed above freezing during storage (Figure 6.10).

Additionally, an external temperature monitor on the plasma storage freezer is helpful in monitoring freezer temperature. These monitors are available with electronic or chart read-outs.

Plastic storage bags may break if mishandled at temperatures below zero. To protect the frozen plasma, wrap the product in plastic bubble wrap prior to freezing. Frozen products should be handled with care!

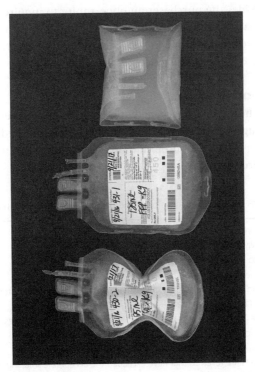

Figure 6.10 Monitoring frozen product storage. The product on the left has a frozen "waist" indentation, while the product on the right contains dead space frozen at the bottom of the bag. The product in the center represents a product that has thawed and re-frozen.

Product Records

A product log is helpful in tracking product use. Donor identification number, donation date, expiration date, volume of product, and final disposition of the unit should be maintained.

Purchasing and Receiving Blood from External Sources

It may be necessary for a veterinary practice to order blood products from outside sources, either exclusively for blood inventory stock or because of an emergency case that consumes all stored blood products during a time when donors are not readily available for blood donation.

It is advisable to establish a client relationship with a reputable veterinary blood bank blood supplier before the need for blood products arises. Communication regarding anticipated need for blood products provides the supplier with valuable information; the supplier can adjust blood collection so that adequate blood supplies are maintained.

This also provides the purchaser an opportunity to inquire as to methods of collection and quality of the donor pool. Additionally, the purchaser may obtain information regarding the suppliers' policies and procedures regarding ordering blood products; examples are listed in Table 6.4.

Receiving Blood Products

Blood products should be unpackaged immediately upon receipt and should be assessed for damage during transport using the guidelines listed in Table 6.5. The product should be placed at appropriate storage temperature and documented as received in the product log.

Table 6.4 Questions related to purchasing blood products from an external vendor

What is the purchase price of the product?

How long does it usually take to get product on a routine basis?

How long will it take to obtain the product for an emergency?

How will the product be packed?

Once packed, how long does the packaging material allow the product optimal storage temperature?

Will overnight shipping be used? What are the associated costs?

Does the delivery route incur extremely hot or extremely cold outside temperatures? Will the packing materials compensate for this?

Are temperature monitoring devices used for the shipping process?

What is the policy if units are received that have exceeded the acceptable shipping temperatures?

What is the policy if the unit is mishandled or lost during shipping?

What will the expiration date(s) of the unit(s) be?

Table 6.5 Assessment of shipped blood products

1. Perform a visual inspection. Is the product damaged in any way? Is there any leaking?
2. Does it appear that the product has been maintained at the proper temperature?
3. Frozen products should arrive frozen!

Preparing Blood Products for Shipment

Blood products should be packaged and shipped in a manner that preserves product integrity. Federal, state, and local guidelines should be reviewed and followed. In some instances, it is necessary to obtain licensure from federal or state agencies prior to shipping blood products.

Product Packaging

Transport containers and packaging procedures should be validated prior to use. These protocols should be periodically monitored to ensure the proper product temperature is maintained throughout the shipping process.

Transport containers should have tight fitting covers and withstand leakage and pressure. Most shippers require that a cooler be shipped with a cardboard box cover. Address labels should be inscribed legibly with indelible ink.

To package blood products for shipping:

1. Obtain a suitable transport container.
2. Within the container, starting from the bottom, layer:
   - coolant
   - absorbent paper
   - product
   - absorbent paper
   - coolant
   - container lid.
3. Secure the coolant lid and exterior box.
4. Attach label.
5. Deliver to shipper.

For whole blood and red cells, the coolant of choice is ice or cold packs, which may be confined in a zip closure plastic bag.

For frozen products, dry ice is the coolant of choice. Dry ice is considered hazardous material as it causes skin burns and releases carbon dioxide as it volatizes. Be sure to notify the shipper that the package contains this hazardous material.

The absorbent paper layers should be capable of containing any leakage within the package. Paper towels, newsprint, or disposable diapers are suitable.

The blood product should also be secured in a zip closure plastic bag in case of accidental damage resulting in subsequent product leakage.

References and Further Reading

Alvedia QuickTEST A+B package insert. Alvedia, Lyon, France.

Alvedia QuickTEST DEA 1.1 package insert. Alvedia, Lyon, France.

Bighignoli B, Niini T, Grahn RA, Pedersen NC, Millon LV, Polli M, Longeri M, Lyons LA. (2007) Cytidine monophospho-N-acetylneuraminic acid hydroxylase (CMAH) mutations associated with the domestic cat AB blood group. *BMC Genet* 8: 27.

Guzman LR, Streeter E, Malandra A. (2016) Comparison of a commercial blood cross-matching kit to the standard laboratory method for establishing blood transfusion compatibility in dogs. *J Vet Emerg Crit Care* 26(2): 262–268.

Hale AS. (2012) Canine blood groups and blood typing. In: *BSAVA Manual of Canine Haematology and Transfusion Medicine*, 2nd edn. Day MJ, Kohn B, eds., pp. 280–283. Gloucester: British Small Animal Veterinary Association.

Kessler RJ, Reese J, Chang D, Seth M, Hale AS, Giger U. (2010) Dog erythrocyte antigens 1.1, 1.2, 3, 4, 7 and *Dal* blood typing and crossmatching by gel column technique. *Vet Clin Pathol* 39(3): 306–316.

Lin M. (2004) Compatibility testing without a centrifuge: the slide Polybrene method. *Transfusion* 44(3): 410–413.

QuickVet® Analyzer Diagnostic System, QuickVet®/RapidVet® Feline Blood Typing Test™ package insert (2015) Scandinavian Micro Biodevices ApS, Farum, Denmark.

RapidVet®-H Canine DEA 1.1 package insert (2014) dmslaboratories, inc., Flemington, NJ.

RapidVet®-H Feline Blood package insert (2012) dmslaboratories, inc., Flemington, NJ.

Seth M, Jackson KV, Winzelberg S, Giger U. (2012) Comparison of gel column, card, and cartridge techniques for dog erythrocyte antigen 1.1 blood typing. *Am J Vet Res* 73(2): 213–219.

Spada E, Proverbio D, Baggiani L, Bagnagatti De Giorgi G, Perego R, Ferro E. (2016) Evaluation of an immunochromatographic test for feline AB system blood typing. *J Vet Emerg Crit Care* 26(1): 137–141.

Virginia Tech Animal Laboratory Services (2015) Blood Bank Procedure Manual (unpublished). Virginia Maryland College of Veterinary Medicine.

Chapter 7 Quality Assurance

Introduction

The main goal of a blood bank or transfusion service is to provide a safe transfusion for every patient. Most organizations regulate and monitor activities related to component preparation, storage, and blood administration; thus, the foundation for a quality system is already in place. Quality programs include quality control, quality assurance, and quality improvement, all of which ensure application of quality principles within operational areas. Examining issues related to quality assurance assist in setting high standards of patient care through constant improvement. All aspects of blood banking, transfusion, and patient care can be analyzed and monitored; the challenge is to regulate variables therein.

The Quality Team

Although basic safety policies and procedures should be in place, it is the practical and concise policy and procedure manuals that provide step-by-step detail for every task performed. A committee of devoted staff can define and set goals related to quality assurance of the transfusion service.

The main purpose of the quality team is to identify and monitor quality indicators. Indicators should be devised to analyze work tasks that can be measured or monitored; results obtained through analysis can be used to improve performance or efficiency of the task. Examples of quality indicators related to blood banks are described in Table 7.1.

Practical Transfusion Medicine for the Small Animal Practitioner, Second Edition. Carolyn A. Sink.
© 2017 John Wiley & Sons, Inc. Published 2017 by John Wiley & Sons, Inc.
Companion website: www.wiley.com/go/sink/transfusion

Table 7.1 Quality indicators related to the blood bank

Action	Quality goal
Monitor length of time for 450 ml blood draw	4–10 minutes
Audit product labels	Accurate labeling
Review product usage	Appropriate transfusion therapy
Blood cultures on expired red cell products	Assures aseptic phlebotomy and component preparation technique
Factor VIII assay for cryoprecipitate	Ensures proper component preparation
Review transfusion reactions	Avoid adverse reaction(s)
Verify equipment and temperature checks	Assures that equipment function

Table 7.2 Attributes of an effective record

Legible
Accurate
Transcription date and time
Identity of the author
Coherent, complete and detailed as necessary to convey meaning
Indelible

Records

Records provide a method of communicating with others and documenting information including observations and opinions. The attributes of an effective record can be found in Table 7.2. Any computer records should be validated for accuracy; data should be protected from unauthorized access and inadvertent changes.

Records Related to the Blood Bank

A blood bank or transfusion service should maintain records pertaining to blood donors and blood recipients. Failure to maintain these records could endanger the blood supply, since valuable information regarding donor health status at the time of donation could be lost. Likewise, targeted look-back is facilitated, if necessary. Pertinent laboratory activities in addition of to donor testing are listed in Table 7.3.

As blood and blood components are distributed, a donor log composed of the date the unit of blood was collected, the unit identification, final volume, expiration date, identification of the preparer, and the final disposition of the unit of blood should be maintained.

If blood and blood products are acquired from an outside source, the log should include these units, including the blood bank from which the products were purchased, the date that they were received, the type and identification of the component, and expiration date.

Federal, state, and local guidelines should be consulted and followed for record storage time. If there are no guidelines, 2-year storage for laboratory records is recommended.

Table 7.3 Laboratory-related records

Personnel training records, including hazard and safety training
Blood storage refrigeration and freezer temperature charts
Equipment maintenance records
Reagent vendors
Quality control of reagents
Quality control of donor units
Blood typing and crossmatch results
Transfusion records
Error and accident reports

Table 7.4 Estimating blood product inventory levels

For a 6-month period, collect data of product usage
Evaluate any unusually high usage; exclude value if considered outlier
Optimum stock level per week = 6-month product usage/24 weeks

Table 7.5 Additional considerations for determining blood product inventory levels

Consideration	Rationale
Number of patients, size of the areas serviced by the hospital	Inventory levels
Average weight of recipient	Determines appropriate blood collection system (product volume)
Expiration date of the product	Which anticoagulant-preservative-additive system is used? If product is received from a supplier, what is the average expiration date? What is the product shelf life?
Services offered by the hospital	Emergency, surgery, and oncology centers typically experience high usage

Inventory Management

Blood product inventory management is difficult since use of blood products can be unpredictable and erratic. Blood products are a valuable commodity and every effort should be made to utilize this product efficiently. It is beneficial to devise a plan for the management of blood products so that this resource is used in a timely and efficient manner.

First, the optimal number of stored units should be established. Each stored product should be analyzed to determine the desired inventory level for that product. If specific blood groups of a particular product are needed, stock levels of each blood group should be evaluated separately. A formula for calculating inventory levels can be found in Table 7.4. Additional factors to be considered when determining optimal stock levels of blood product are given in Table 7.5. It may also be useful to institute internal policies with regard to blood products to assist in inventory management (Table 7.6). These policies should be communicated to all staff members who may transfuse blood products.

Table 7.6 Practical methods to control product usage

Method	Desired result
Arrange products in the refrigerator and freezer so that the oldest unit will be pulled first	This will make using the oldest unit convenient and optimize product usage
Establish ordering guidelines	Make sure each clinician knows and understands the goals of component therapy and that once the order is given to transfuse, the product will be removed from storage and prepared for immediate transfusion
Develop procedures for issuing blood components	Specify how many units may be prepared for one patient at a given time
Develop procedures for obtaining products when stock levels are diminished	Assures adequate inventory is maintained

References and Further Reading

Motschman TL, Jett BW, Wilkinson SL. (2014) Quality management systems: theory and practice. In: *American Association of Blood Banks Technical Manual*, 18th edn., pp. 39–64. Bethesda, MD: American Association of Blood Banks.

Food and Drug Administration (FDA) (1995) Guideline for Quality Assurance in Blood Establishments. Available at: www.fda.gov/downloads/BiologicsBloodVaccines/Guidance ComplianceRegulatoryInformation/Guidances/Blood/UCM164981.pdf

World Health Organization (WHO) (1993) Guidelines for quality assurance programmes for blood transfusion services. Available at: http://apps.who.int/iris/handle/10665/41752

Index